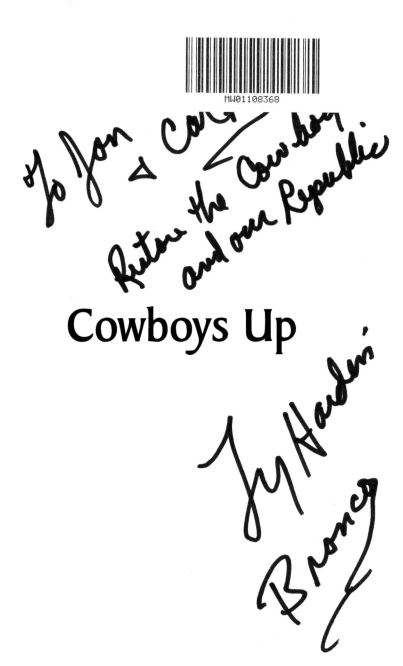

To Jon & Cara
Return the Cowboy
and our Republic

Cowboys Up

Jy Harden
Bronco

Cowboys Up:

"Armageddon"

Ty Hardin

To order additional copies of this book, contact:
Xlibris Corporation
1-888-795-4274
www.Xlibris.com
Orders@Xlibris.com
54497

Contents

Foreword

WELL, I HAVE gone and done it. I'm one of the few TV cowboys left in the game; and *Cowboy Up* is my last tribute and praise to my heroes of the silver screen – Roy, Gene, and Hoppy who were my role models as I was growing up. The days of cowboys and Indians are long gone, and pride in our heritage and Christian values have left the silver screen. Our kids have very little connection to our history as it has been purposely omitted from their young experience by the new age capitalists. My book is a tragedy in process as we sit back and watch the moral decay of our nation and our Christian values being dumped into the sewers of America. You might say I'm bitter, but you would be wrong. I'm embarrassed to be so naive to think freedom doesn't come at a price. Diligence and justice must prevail, and both have been trashed by our pastors and so-called elected representatives in our government. The Congress almost changed their loyalties to support the people with their votes, but money and intimidation won out. These gutless frauds who pretend to represent the interests of the people have now provoked the wrath of God upon themselves, and their mentors winning them a special place in hell. The show is not over, and America is waking up. I hope we are not too late for us to see those globalists fry in hell. They may be able to fool the flocks, but they damn sure cannot fool our Creator God. May God have mercy on their miserable souls!

Ty Hardin

Introduction

*S*EEK AND YE shall find. The world events now being presently played out before a world audience of dumb-down, brain-dead humanity – addicted to lusting after temporal, worldly, material goodies – have become openly receptive to the megamedia microprocessing of their minds. They have lost their God awareness and creative qualities to chasing the almighty dollar while ignoring their God-given talents of expressing original thought. They have become puppets to a cleverly contrived, media-hyped world that has stolen their minds, imaginations, and desires in seeking original thought. They have allowed themselves to be taxed and raped of their dignity and property. They have reduced themselves into a herd of humanity, entrenched in mimicking the rhetoric of their self-inflicted role models from Hollywood. They have become consistent seekers of mindless entertainment, keeping their minds entertained and from having to face reality that their lives and nation are being reduced into a herd of lemmings. The entertainment icons have carefully selected their story plots using sex, violence, and graphic visuals to lull the world's populations into complacent herds of the blind leading the blind.

Humanity has lost its ability to create and sustain creative freethinking society. They are preoccupied in surviving in the new age mentality controlled by the international globalists. Their media control has affected our children's minds who can no longer be taught the values of our freedoms.

Our once-enlightened, God-fearing societies have been programmed into a gullible herd of new age mummies. How in God's name can we not question the government's rhetoric that proclaimed two jetliners took down three steel buildings in their tracks and turn them into toxic powder in ten minutes? As an electrical engineer, I know for a fact what it takes if they were not rigged to collapse into dust and who did it. Where are all those weapons of mass destruction, Bush? But blame Bush, where are the God-loving Christians whose God demands that only the "truth shall set you free"? When will they step up to the plate and force their government to be accountable? Are we all too busy struggling to make ends meet to address the real threat to our freedoms, a government gone amuck? Is our billion-dollar American war machine being used to support a globalist agenda to gain total control over all earth resources? Our young soldiers are being finely tuned to take military control over the entire world. It appears we now have a standing army stationed throughout the world that is now the most lethal force in the world. It certainly is not my desire to own the oil reserves in Iran or Iraq when we need to get off oil dependency. The real problem is finding enemies to feed their military machine and support their agenda of culling world populations. It appears they need to sustain the world's fear and respect for their massive military force. They don't have any obvious enemies except a few that they have created with aggressive actions against the Arab nations, sitting on the world's largest oil reserves. We all are aware the world has a real problem of overpopulation and pollution, stressing out all life on the planet. I just shopped at our mall, and it was packed with "implants."

Eighty percent of the shoppers were of foreign origin. Most of them were speaking a foreign language. All had at least two kids and more on the way. I mean, the floodgates have been opened to foreigners and with no regulations being enforced. My great-grandparents came from England and took the land away from the Indians, and now we are giving it back to Asians and Europeans. It seems we built this nation for the globalists' agenda so they can use our army and gold to take over the world. Do you think for one moment the bankers aren't enjoying watching the lemmings being duped into believing we have a world full of terrorists who hate our freedoms? Boy, I had no idea how gullible and docile our people have become to let their government destroy our love and respect for all God's creations. They are using our taxed dollars and our kids to finance and man their international wars for world control. It must be exciting for those globalists to dream up such misery and strife for the inhabitants of our planet. I wonder what disease or plague they will conjugate up next to augment their dreams of a globalist community. Since World War II, we haven't won a single encounter with their trumped-up terrorist nations. Did you ever wonder why none of their wars has ended with a decisive victory? Vietnam, Korea, Iraq, and soon Iran are examples of our armies continual fighting for globalists' agenda. What about all our young men who are being sacrificed? Just kids looking for opportunities in life, I was on of them when I joined to fight in Korea. I was a young kid who believed it was honorable and patriotic to fight for the government's agenda. I had no clue that 33,731kids died in Korea for the globalists' agenda.

Our globalists have managed to divide the world, causing every nation in the world to be our enemy or our coconspirator. It doesn't surprise me seeing nations now banding together to protect themselves from our evil intentions. It is quite obvious we, the American people, are not calling the shots. Truth is, the government is not under the control of the people, and we have no voice in the performance of the new age government. Our vote is a mockery to our intelligence as we all know there is no difference among the candidates. Politics is business as usual. How much hostility and animosity have we created throughout the world? I did travel the world over, working in foreign films, enjoying respect from all nations as an American cowboy actor, who loved his Christian values.

On June 4, 1963, an attempt was made by President Kennedy to strip the Federal Reserve Bank of its power to create, print, and distribute our paper money. Executive Order 11110, still on the books in Congress, returned the authority and power to the U.S. government as per the Constitution to print and regulate our currency. The elected officials and freethinkers were all aware that President Kennedy was terminated because he was restoring a gold-backed U.S. dollar. You see, that act would have stopped the globalists' banks from inflating and creating wealth out of thin air as the dollar would have to evaluate against silver or gold stored in Fort Knox. Restoring gold- and silver-backed currency negated their powers of creating money out of thin air. (Read murderers of President Kennedy.) The globalists have nothing but contempt for our belief in God. Life evolves and its origin is a mystery; you live and die.

They enjoy belittling Christians for their belief in a fictitious fairy tale that happened hundreds of years ago. What could an event that happened over two thousand years ago have an impact on today's events? They live with no allegiances as they live in a temporal existence that bears no real purpose except the pleasures they derive from personal gains. The elite globalists enjoy patronizing the Christians as they are all peace lovers and are no real threat to their world agenda. They keep them under control with laws that keep them from getting evolved in government. Intimidation is used on all churches that don't play ball – stay out of politics and all government affairs, or pay taxes.

Where are our staunch leaders of our nation? These professing ambassadors of God have all fallen prey to global money system as they do not want to lose their tax-free status from speaking out against banking usury as Jesus did. (Owe no man anything.) We, the people, have lost our voice and freedoms as we are a nation submerged in debt to the world bankers. Our spiritual leaders are silent, sitting by and watching our nation being subdued into total financial slavery. The forces of evil are being prepared for a resurrection of freedom as the truth is coming out, and men are getting desperate to survive in our failing economy. Every man knows in his heart where the problem lies. They all can see that the bankers have stolen all our natural resources, and the government is bailing them out with their bogus printing presses. We oldies remember when a nickel bought a Coke and a candy bar. We are living in bondage to our debt, creature comforts, and inflated economy. The chickens are coming home to roost as the globalists take our nation.

I place the real blame on complacent Christians that have ignored and compromised their Christian values and freedoms for personal gains into the bankers' commercial world. It is called render-unto-Caesar-what-is-Caesar's syndrome. Americans no longer take the responsibility of their actions to see that their governments reflect and obey the values God had laid down in his constitution to govern his people. We have become divided as Americans into bickering Republicans and Democrats and forgetting we all should be constitutionalists? Where are the minutemen? Where are the Bible thumpers who follow God's commandments? We are that "one nation under God," a myth of the past as we are enslaved into the sin of usury. We Americans should be voting for a man best suited for the job, not a party representative who mimics personal interests of the elites that put him into office. Wake up, Christians, satanic forces have divided God's chosen nation that was and has been blessed by him and commissioned to be a guiding example unto the world. We believers in Christ have been commissioned by God to spread Christianity throughout his world. We no longer practice what we preach. Do you not see that God no longer can bless this nation and has to give it up to reap the consequences of our greed and disobedience to God. We are a morally corrupted nation whose godly endowed values and principles have been squandered and ignored. We are now in a self-destructing mode with greed and evil being projecting in our foreign policies. The free world is uniting against us as they band together to prevent NATO from taking away their sovereignty. God cannot bless a nation intent on destroying creation.

Can you not see that this nation has compromised all its godly principles? (You shall put no other gods before me.) God is surely weeping as he witnesses the rejection of his love and wisdom that could restore prosperity to our land. "What you sow you shall reap." *We* have created the maximum fear for mankind, an atomic holocaust, our gift to mankind. What a great legacy for our children. We have the capability to destroying totally all humanity on this planet. We are the only nation that has expressed our willingness to use our atomic bombs on any nation that dares to oppose our one-world order. We have become a mockery to God's laws and sanctity of life as we show no concern for his creation. Can you imagine, for one minute, how you would feel if someone you created to love was about to destroy the very creation you built for him to enjoy and prosper? Can you not see that this evil will force the wrath of God upon us? Will the Holy Spirit intervene and save us from ourselves? Why should it? What have we done to propagate peace and love between our fellow mankind? We have been endowed by God with free volition to worship our God from a willing heart and free soul. He had no intentions of creating a world of puppets to serve him in fear and obedience. He desires a spiritual bond with his creation and works his will through the exercise of our free volition. That brings glory to his name and gives him great pleasure to feel the return of his love with expressions that reflects unconditional agape love. It excites God seeing us bringing glory to his name as it does when my wife cooks up a great meal for me. We believers have been given the spiritual responsibility of presenting his love and hope to the lost world.

The few spiritual leaders left in our society are no longer a force in his church (body of Christ) as they have been fragmented into denominations, teaching their own form of his Bible. A few serious-minded, intelligent, gifted, godly men who have dared to speak out on the issues of today are being silenced by intimidation, ridicule, and fear of harm. Events presently are being played out on the world stage reflect the complete destruction of all free societies worldwide. We ignore the fact that we are dealing with certain societies that are fatalists and have no fear of death. If given the opportunity, provoked excessively, they would and could destroy our world with no regrets. Is that what happened to Mars?

Our globalist world ambitions could set off a world holocaust that could make Hitler's deeds look like a picnic. There is a group of people I refer to who would welcome an opportunity to martyr their lives to serve their god. This is a future event we cannot afford to ignore as the globalists have created more enemies worldwide than they realize. These nations are keenly aware of our senseless culling of humanity, and you can be rest assured they are going to find every means available to survive at all costs. They read the event of today and see the devastation we are bringing upon their lands and people with our armies, global warming, and rampant release of new incurable diseases (AIDS, papilloma, chlamydia) in their societies. The world societies are fully aware of the globalists' intentions to cull the world populations and possess total control over all natural resources. You can be assured the world is not asleep and are preparing for our attacks on their sovereign nations.

The events preceding the destruction of our earth are now in full bloom, along with the return of Jesus Christ for those who choose to believe in our Bible. Why? Because the destruction of our present society is certain, and the forces of evil are in place and fully implemented to take domination over all the earth and the forces of God. This agenda has been well prepared, and nothing is left for chance. Ever since the bombing of Japan after we were winning the war, the world has witnessed our leaders' true hypocrisy and godless nature from the senseless killing of Japanese civilians with atrocity that could have been just a demonstration. We introduced maximum fear into the world with that atomic bomb. The point of no return has been reached as predicted in God's Word. Astronomical changes are evident in every facet of life on God's planet. We all live with the fear that some nation will instigate an atomic holocaust. We look to our government for our protection, but they are the culprits that are bringing the wrath of God down on us. (To whom much is given much is expected.) It is not the world that is in disobedience to God. It is our nation and allies that God has blessed and set up to be his body of Christ on earth. Lusting after temporal goodies and worldly treasures has jeopardized our earthly security. All societies have been infiltrated by the forces of evil, the World Bankers. Will they succeed? That, my dear readers, is solely in the hands of the living God. We are all but temporal inhabitants living on his earth, under his control, so live with it. This earth is his creation, and he alone sustains and maintains controls over all his inhabitants. God will prevail even if mankind would self-destruct.

You need to accept and know the truth "as the truth shall set you free." This book is designed and dedicated to bringing your mind to a spiritual awareness as it is revealed and documented in the archives of his Bible. No one said truth had to be a beautiful picture. What I would like to know is where are his godly, fearless, patriotic men we call his body on earth? Are they ignoring the fact that the forces of evil are boldly moving to destroy God's kingdom on earth. Where was the body of Christ when we bombed Hiroshima? Why haven't they stepped forward to stop this insanity of greed and contempt for God's creation that inevitably will bring on the destruction of our planet? Evil men, possessed by satanic forces, are now capable of destroying all life on our planet. Most governments worldwide are now brain-dead humanoids that dance to the tune of the world bankers. There are the emissaries of satanic behind all types of atrocities against humanity.

The pressure of living day by day in a usury of society, submerged in financial bondage, is driving our populations into committing all forms of crimes against our society, just to feed their families. The world is being stressed out, falling apart, getting ready to implode in crime and killing. That action will play right into the hands of the elites that want a reason to declare their martial law and bring our nation under the control of their homeland security. You think that's far-fetched? What is Homeland Security all about? I thought we had a local police force that answered to the people, not to a handful of globalists. Who instigated it, criminal cowards with evil intentions? What was their purpose? Certainly not to protect the nation.

Homeland security is set up to protect the criminals in government from the massive patriots who are beginning to appear as they see through the lies and deceit from the government stooges. The politicians have sold out our constitutional freedoms to the global bankers who have been granted power of government to perfect their globalists' agenda. Their next action is to enact martial law after their next-planned disaster. My gut feeling is they will stage another false 9/11 to kill off few million defenseless eaters. I will give them credit to move the masses to support their martial law. You see, I first came to California. I worked as an engineer at Douglas Aircraft Company in Santa Monica. I worked on suppressors for the DC-8 Conway engines in 1974. No thinking engineer could validate the concept that a four-engine airplane could vaporize a steel-structured building. That just isn't possible. Can you imagine how many engineers in America are sitting on their butts, accepting the government lies, knowing full well that their nation is under attack from some hidden force? They know as I do that gasoline can't generate enough heat to melt steel beams and cause buildings to implode into a heap of ashes. It was an inside job, poorly executed and badly acted. With control of media, the globalists were able to cover up their evil atrocities and get the nation to support their global agenda

Enough doom and gloom as only a few of you believe what this cowboy has to say. Let's discuss God's nature of projecting agape love toward all his creation. He requires in his Word for creation to live peacefully on his planet. He rules creation only by his divine nature of love that demands peaceful solutions.

Your God can only expresses himself through his divine love as shown to us by the life Jesus Christ had on earth. Unconditional love, in return, to our God is the only means that mankind has to enjoying a peaceful and prosperous existence on his planet. All the hell that we bring upon ourselves can be attributed to our rebellious nature of being like the Most High. Our dilemma is in trying to understand the nature of God's love and how to express it in our daily lives. Being a loving God, he has given his creations free volition to map out their own destiny. Sure, we evolved from cavemen and maybe out of trees, but our divine nature is and always has been to be connected to our creator. That fact has always existed as it is witnessed in the archives of images left in caves and rock walls. Mankind has always perceived to have a creator. It's built into his very nature. There are a lot of gods in history that mankind has created and worshiped. He has revealed to me and millions of believers that God entered into humanity in the person of Jesus Christ. I am convinced by his teachings and the work of the Holy Spirit that he is our sole creator. Everything has perfection and meaning and is perfectly adaptable to live in harmony with our environment and belief systems.

If you live with a limited recognition of God that has to conform to your mental condition of independence, then you negate a relationship with your creator. He enjoys being the object of your affections. It is a mental condition we perfect by having a spirit-filled relationship with our God through our Lord, Jesus Christ. Unfortunately, his believers are not fully dedicated to seeking his will for their lives.

That is the tragic condition of the church today. Christians should be uniting to heal our land, not segmented into ineffective small groups trying to survive effectively in a deteriorating society. Do you think for one moment Jesus enjoys seeing his body of believers scrapping the bottom of the barrel to forge a living? Squabbling over doctrinal differences when his nation faces moral collapse? What will it take to bring his believers together to face the real threat to our nation – the godless heathen that are in control of our government and national debt? We, the chosen people of God, are a mockery to his name as we have forsaken our Lord in pursuit of the almighty dollar. Look at the all-seeing-eye emblem on their dollar, smiling at your ignorance. With a mockery directed at you, it says, "In God we trust." Living with financial slavery has come home to rouse as our nation is going under. You may think you have salvation from eternal death, but you're living in pure hell on earth for your transgressions. The hell this nation is presently going through will make the Great Depression look like a picnic. We have lost our first love and are following after temporal, earthly rewards that God provided for man to enjoy, not worship. Is it the divine nature of mankind to live like the Most High? We like being kings in our own right and enjoy feeling we have total control of our destiny. Our God image has been limited and has to conform to our egos. When we get closer to death, we can always alter our thinking and become better Christians, right? You realize, of course, you are doing God an injustice as you have become a god by making God conform to your belief system. If you choose that course for your life, then you stand in defiance to God.

You will then reap the consequences of a life in chaos, vacillating through the human experience with no mental stability, inner loneliness, and meaningless wondering on a hostile earth. Jesus paid the ultimate price to set an example of a spirit-filled life. Could he expect anything less from his flock? Why are we chasing temporal, earthly gains that can never satisfy the soul that's separate from its creator? Did you ever ask yourself "where is the proof that God exists"? Why has he not revealed himself to his creation in physical form? Can a creative force that hung the universe not do what he wants to do? Could your God be a spirit and talk through the writers of his scriptures to you? Have you never been inspired to reach for a higher knowledge and awareness? Do you not desire to believe you were created for a divine purpose, or do you prefer to remain a wondering vagabond, trying to find reality and purpose for your life? The Bible defines the essence of God's Word as written by men who were inspired and in tune with the spirit of God. Peter was rebellious but never questioned *who Jesus was.* Have you lived your life and never been inspired by God? Have you never felt the hands of God on your life as you have traveled through your life's experiences? Do your eyes not witness the massiveness and beauty of his creation? Does not all creation have an origin that has been given a divine purpose? The birds, insects, animals – all have meaning and purpose created within their beings. Some omnipotent, omnipresent, omniscient force has started the whole ball game going and keeps it moving at a regular pace despite our rebellious nature. Let's get real, let God be God and allow him to be involved in all our lives.

Think for a second on the magnitude of perfection and the force it takes to keep all the planets in the universe in line to prevent a universal holocaust. Is an asteroid headed your way? We take creation for granted, not realizing we are only a small part of a great, magnificent expression of a loving God's imagination. We are all aware nothing happens by chance, and there is finite order in all creation. You are a unique person, and God will not create another you on this planet? You alone can direct your thoughts and accept his son Jesus as God's expression of love directed right at you. Don't allow your mind to become confused and let it think you don't have divine purpose for your life. Get involved with like-minded believers, people who allow God to direct their lives through prayer and inspiration. It's in your life's interests to elevate your thinking, belief system, and faith to believe there is a Creator God who holds the very purpose for your life in his hands. You may never know it until you ask for guidance and vision. If you do, then take on confidence and know your life is on the path to enlightenment. This is an instinctive quality God establishes in all his believers. We don't have to live without hope, and we can enjoy inner peace with God that programs our minds to rest in confidence that he is a God of his Word. What a small sacrifice we pay to live with eternal peace, enjoying life with our mind at peace with our souls. We stop wandering aimlessly over the planet, looking for something to fill that hole in our heart and soul. Boy, have I been there, and it's not pretty. Believers become empowered of God and enjoy a connection with the omnipotent force of the Creator God. Your life takes on a godly appearance.

What purpose would life serve if there was no meaning in all creation? Animals seem to have no problem fulfilling their purpose for existence as it is built into their instinctive qualities from their very birth. We are also included in that program as it is built into our natures as well. It is an instinctive quality to seek, know, and analyze God's purpose for our lives. We seem to desire to analyze every thing we do and think, forgetting sometimes we could be reacting to an inner inspiration that comes from a divine source. I hear "The devil made me do it" and not as often "God made me do it." I don't think man is serving multiple interests even though there may be many options on the table. This is where our belief systems steps in and helps us choose the direction God would have us go. I believe that God directs our paths in this life only when we choose to gave him that responsibility. You see, God is working within me both to will and do his good pleasure. That, my dear readers, is active faith at work. Let's think just for one second at the alternative. Let's say, for an extreme example, you're one of those globalists that are hell-bent on controlling God's world. What if you were to gain this world but lost your eternal soul? How can life be profitable if you lose the very purpose for existence? Well, you say, you just don't believe in eternal life. Right, then what is this show all about?

Just someone's hair-brained idea of a joke? Why go to all that trouble of fulfilling your egos and having a lustful life and end up just dead meat? Is someone playing a trick on us, giving us a desire without a solution? Why does my mind conceive the existence of an eternal God if it is an illusion? There has to be some source as my life is not an illusion.

It all boils down to belief. I believe if my mind is capable of conceiving eternal life, then it could be valid and then millions of Christians worldwide are not disillusioned or deceived into living with eternal hope. If this whole concept is somebody's great farce, then this is the greatest deceit ever perpetuated on the human herd. It is a lot of truths and garbage thrown into ancient manuscript that has deceived mankind for hundreds of years. The brilliance of these writers is beyond anything I could have ever imagined. The one verse that works for me is "what if we gain the *whole world* and lose our own *souls* to *hell*?" Cowboys, the world we live in will exist with or without our consent. It's comforting and essential to enjoy a belief system that works for you, that lifts your spirits, and that places eternal hope within your life. What do I have to lose that isn't offset with what I have to gain? I know God's Word, and I have found comfort and enjoyment being obedient to his Word. Your creator offers you eternal life in the form of his son, who died in your place on the cross to redeem you from the penalty of sin and eternal death of your soul (wages of sin is death). Tell me, how would you communicate with your creator if you desired to have fellowship with him? It would have to be on some mutual level of communication, right? The mind recognizes that all physical life on earth is terminal; however, the soul-mind desires the possibility of internal life. Its instinct must have been created within our awareness by design. The struggles we have within are only satisfied when we exercise our positive belief system that includes the origin of life. Eternal hope is the cornerstone for the Christian faith. Hope gives our lives the added dimension of eternal peace.

Our faith grants us an internal freedom from anxiety and strife from the chaotic world we live in. Man without his God-centered belief system struggles daily, looking and seeking for a purpose in his life. That discontentment is the root of all anxiety that initiates wars, strife, and chaos that could easily be the demise for all creation. Mankind has always been restless and discontented within his life when he is separated from a belief in his Creator God. That void is the power that drives evil man into a self-destructive mode of seeking power over all creation. That is where humanity is today. Evil men looking for gratification with power over all God's creation by printing a false god – money. God counters with "Come unto me all ye that are heavy laden, and I will grant you peace." What a powerful statement Jesus made to all who take him at his Word. His world is now being ruled by fatalistic, desperate men who look at life as a temporal experience. They live without eternal hope and a desire to cram all the living they can into the few years of existence. A life without God awareness is an empty life without eternal hope. Hope is man's mind contemplating a better future for his life. Hope also offers his life the added dimension of a purpose to his existence. I now face every day the reality that I am a short-timer on his planet as I am seventy-eight years young. My faith in my God has defined the purpose for my life and a reality to eternal life. It has added a peaceful existence into my life that has added health and years to my life. It has given me a desire and purpose to live by helping others find the way into eternal contentment. Death holds no dominion over me, and if God chooses to take me home tomorrow, I am packed and ready.

All that materialistic security the globalists have acquired from printing paper wealth will not grant them a pass into eternity when they are called to cross over into the spiritual world. They will need a godly approval from the gatekeeper. Their material gains are no down payment for a seat in his kingdom. This world may offer those globalists a false sense of importance and security, but they all face physical death and will have to deal with the possibility of dealing with their souls subject to eternal hell. What if all those disillusioned Christians are right, globalists?

Where are you now with all your financial security? What irks me is these men profess to have intelligence and are attempting to take over all God's creation. The world doesn't belong to them, and their bogus money can't buy it. Christian men and women built this great American society and dedicated it to their God. Why are they so blind as to try and take control of God's property and cull out his believers, knowing they just might have to reap the full wrath of that living God? Is their real problem in having to accept the sovereignty of Jesus Christ as their Lord and Savior? You accept death. Just look at the rewards, eternal peace within and a permanent residence secured in his heaven. Why would an atheistic globalist seek to enjoy a temporal existence on earth with his money and power and totally neglect the possible existence of his eternal soul? Why would he choose to live without eternal hope in exchange for the senseless existence one has on earth without eternal hope? All your aspirations are of no consequence when it all ends up in a heap of ashes. A creator wouldn't create a life without divine purpose, and pursuit of *money* is bad investment.

The super elites live in an isolated world of their own making. They have no contact with the real world but live in fear of exposure to their aspirations of world control. They have bodyguards and castles for protection from the world around them. They are conscious of their evil intentions for the world and do not want that exposure to the masses. It has been well documented that they have committed multiple atrocities against the human race. Their evil desires of total control of God's creation have forced them to commit gross atrocities against all God's creation. The atomic bombs and deadly bugs are their evil contribution to mankind. Believe me, they won't escape the judgment of the living God who won't sit around, watching his creation being destroyed by these evil men much longer. They can't escape his judgment even though they are presently trying to find a means to live life forever. The scary part is that they have neither conscience nor remorse for the atrocities they have committed against God's creation. One that irks me is that the restless soul wanders in an empty vacuum, seeking a god that approves of his evil deeds. Satanic worship is becoming very predominant in that society today. That satisfies his warped mind and ignores his soul's desires to connect with its Creator God.

Look at the condition of our world today as it is now being run by the godless globalists. Life is in chaos with families who are homeless, dollar values being dumped, jobs gone south, food shortages coming in, and a society that is bankrupted. Our previous vision of peace and equality for mankind is now a myth. Our once-godly nation is now on the verge of total spiritual and financial collapse.

Our elite rulers have totally ignored creation as if it never existed. Global warming and famines are their legacy as they focus on how they will take total control over the affairs of mankind without being exposed. Fear of failure possesses their souls as they are competing with an omnipotent force – God – who has expressed ultimate patience with these ignorant globalists who are now growing thin. There is a silent beast waiting in the shadows, ready to expose the traitors in government to the masses. They will need a real advanced 9/11 to get this nation behind their bid for a one-world order. And we know they are desperate people and will perform desperate deeds. Globalists are now setting up plans to take an aggressive action against Iran that will throw China and Russia into the game. They need oil too, and the world is starting to get the picture that we are after all the world's natural resources when we set up so-called terrorists attacks against our nation. Nobody told me what Iraq wanted from their attack on our three old skyscrapers. We don't have any of their people in our prisons, and we sure don't have any gold to give them. Maybe someday, we will know the truth on how they knocked down three old skyscrapers with two airplanes. I don't buy they-hate-our-freedoms crap, enough to martyr themselves.

Do you think for one moment God is going to sit back and watch his creation go up in smoke? Destroyed by a handful of desperate globalists who have no respect of his creation? I'm sure God will inspire the body of Christ to fill in the gaps of leadership in his political arena. God enjoys rising up Christian patriots to meet the challenges of today. He knows he will receive the glory from his believers.

A soul that is not grounded in God's Word is lost and tormented, destined to self-destruct. I have watched satanic forces move into the film industry, take over most of the film production, and turn the industry into a tool for secular humanism that mocks the existence of God. The modern film producers of today are mostly Zionists who have rejected the claims of Jesus and fill their troubled souls with making worldly films filled with illicit sex, godless plots that downgrade our Christian values and mock his principles. My once-great film industry brought hope, feelings, and inspired entertainment to our world and especially our children, our future masses. Today, it contaminates our children's minds with secular garbage, subhuman story plots, and satanic-debauch dialogue that shows no respect for our godly values and principles that inspired our children into divine leadership in the world.

They have totally eliminated a godly influence in their secular films with the help of their puppets in the Washington and American Civil Liberties Union (ACLU), which has taken our God out of our schools and public places. Where are our Christian warriors in the churches when the government stole the minds of our children? I remember making good patriot films like *PT 109*. Merrill's Marauders and others had our viewers feeling good about our nation, our freedoms, and the world we lived in. We are now a depressed nation living on drugs, paying usury, and chasing the almighty dollar. Many call upon his name, fill the churches, but he knows them not as they give lip service without commitment and dedication. His light still flickers for a few that God has separated to stand fast in these last days of freedom. You will stand with God or live under fear.

The Christ of our Bible will not share a place in your life with Satan. You can't expect evil and good to coexist for control of your life. Pick today who you will serve and who will have control over your thoughts and actions. Sure, you will slip and fall, but your Lord is compassionate and understanding and will not allow you to be tempted above what you are not able to handle. I have chosen God to join me.

A new breed of filmmakers have taken over Hollywood's productions and are an abomination to God. These producers live as parasites feeding off our immature children, forming their minds with sick plots, profanity, illicit sex, and depressing story lines supporting their one-world agenda. The new role models for our children are toys to their agenda of dummying down our children. They are focused on sex, violence, admiration for wealth, and lavished living styles. Their minds are being programmed, centered on violence and sexual expressions that form patterns in young lives that will render them godless and helpless in the new world of haves and have-nots. They will not be able to cope in this new age and are prime candidates for a miserable life. They are victims of the new age mentality, struggling for opportunity and being content with nothing. There are no longer any Christian role models in the industry to pattern their lives after. The future of our nation is in the hands of our children, and if we don't bring them up in the ways of the Lord, they will be pawns in the globalists' agenda. These new age film producers are making films laced with sex, profanity, and sick plots aimed at destroying any godly traits and values that might have been planted in their subconscious minds by exposure to Christianity or godly parents.

I realize my lost and confused state when I ended up in a Spanish prison for dealing drugs. God got my attention, and Franco (Spain's dictator) listened to my repentance and set me free in Gibraltar in four days. You see, I was living in denial as I thought I could be a Christian and live a debauched existence with money and prestige the focus of my affections. I had a sad awakening. They had put me in the cell with all the homosexuals where I would be safe. They were harmless as homosexuals, and generally, they were pacifists. It was against the law in Franco's Spain. I was petrified and couldn't sleep for three days. Franco, after finding out I was in his prison, released me and took me to Málaga and put me on the boat to Gibraltar. I not only got a wake-up call but got out of a scary place, and God restored my faith in Jesus as my Lord and Savior. I rededicated my life to God and haven't turned back to Satanism again. I returned to the States after my son Bobby rescued me from jail from Texas and brought me some money to start kicking my life all over. As I look back at that experience, it was a major turning point in my life. Sure, I had some rough times since, but I haven't forsaken my calling. This book will be my last offering to my public service and exposure. I am having a fit trying to find my notch in the writer's kingdom. "Seek and you shall find," my God has said, and that has been my incentive to forge ahead with this book, seeking to serve my God with the remaining part of my life. I have worked and struggled for seventy-eight years of living on this planet, and I am now ready to retire and seek my final adventure with my God. I am presently seeking a little wisdom in identifying myself with God's purpose for these last years of my life.

The evidence of his agape love is all around me, but I have failed in the past to look at it with his spiritual eyes. I am still struggling with my personal inner drives and have failed to give God proper credit for any of my success in my past life as I see it as wasted time. I have now accepted my existence as a natural function of the perpetual life existence we all have on this planet. One is in physical form and the other in the spiritual nature living in harmony with laws set down by God. However, I feel that nothing is forever, and we live on a short fuse, engaged in the process of propagating and terminating life on this planet along with establishing our spiritual destiny in eternity. Mankind, without a faith in the living God, is constantly in the process of self-destructing his life. He indulges in escapisms such as drugs, temporal enjoyments, war games, and gorging his gut with contaminated foods. He lives with an obvious expression of termination and self-destruction with little or no concern for the future of his life as he accepts futility for a lifestyle as the body winds up in the grave. Mankind as a whole has lost respect for himself and the human race. This condition is the direct outcome of ignoring the creative force of a living God. The self-programmed mind of the agnostic does not hold to the concept that we reap what we have sown as they become fatalists and can't change their fate. The world is their playground, and they are the gods of their world. Their values vacillate from day to day by the whims of time. They seek purpose for life in all the wrong places. Power, sex, greed, overindulgence, self-adulation, and drugs are the last resort of being totally discontent with life.

The Mature Life

GLOBAL WARMING ALONE will eliminate life on our planet as it is being ignored by the globalists as fear plays into their hands. We sit around and do nothing about it. We earthlings are so complacent and ignorant to the amount of toxic imbalance we are developing and depositing upon our earth. We allow greedy politicians to control our lives as long as they offer us creature comforts to escape the reality of our desperate condition. Car emissions alone, if we don't stop using fossil fuels, will eventually eliminate all life on this planet. That is trivial compared to what a few well-placed atomic bombs will do our civilization on earth. It will create a lethal haze of toxic fallout over earth that has a life span of enough years to wipe out all civilizations.

I'm not standing in judgment of religious concepts or belief systems in this diverse world, that's God's duty and responsibility; but where are all our intellectual, rational freethinkers of our world who have great knowledge of the history of mankind and his shortcomings? Can they not see what is going on today? Has the media, controlled by the world globalists, stamped out all free speech and silenced the freethinkers? Our minds have been warped and channeled into ignoring creation, losing respect for ourselves, and allowing our minds to dwell on our gift's pride on understanding the basic qualities of our Creator God. We believers in freethinking and free expression have become lemmings that will remain asleep in our complacency and church surroundings while enjoying our creature comforts, living by the concept of "let God sort this out." We shall reap what we have sowed. Ignorance to God's Word is no excuse.

It's not my responsibility to pass judgment on to the events of this world, but when the head of state is invited over to speak, the lest he should expect is to be treated with dignity and respect for his position of president of a sovereign nation. The judgment of that man I'll leave onto the hands of the Creator and his actions. I won't be trapped into senseless arguments with men who live with blinders and have been programmed to believe our government's rhetoric. I do know and recognize we are witnessing the rapid deterioration of our society both morally and financially.

All our core values that built this great nation were rooted in Christianity. That belief system has brought our nation prosperity and respect. We portrayed a sense of kindness and fairness toward all mankind worldwide. We have led the world by example up to now. The greed of our elite bankers has destroyed our creditability in the world with usury that has bankrupted our people along with many others. I remember well when I traveled the world over, making films overseas that we were revered and loved by all. We Americans were welcomed to all parts of the world, and we were treated with respect as we were not a threat to anyone. We have lost that position as we are now envied and despised in many parts of this world. Our population's greedy entrepreneurs are now spending billions on drugs, entertainments, and self-indulgence to escape the reality of mankind's responsibility to God for his life, liberty, and prosperity. We have now become the most hated and envied nation in the world. We have evolved into a self-serving society that is submerged in self-indulgence, ignoring creation and focusing on temporal earthly goodies as the object of our affections. He who dies with the most goodies has won a place in the sun is now our standard for life. As we now faced with the real possibility of annihilating all life on our planet, maybe it's time we, the rulers of this nation, take a little interest in the caliber of representatives we put in Washington. We need to focus our energies on finding the means to live peacefully on God's planet and with all its inhabitants. We have built our military bases in 157 sovereign countries with 325,000 troops in them. Who are they protecting?

We have a total of 737 bases on foreign soils that control 2,202,735 hectares of 130 foreign nations. We are a bankrupt nation living off the bankers' usury, but we spend 626 billion U.S. dollars a year of our hard-earned tax money to maintain our army's personnel in those occupied bases. That action secures private corporate world of raping all the natural resources from those sovereign nations while intimidating them with our troops. Do you think for one minute we do not maintain total control over all the world's populations and all natural resources needed to sustain life on godforsaken planet? Read all the figures for yourself and know well that nothing in this world happens by chance. The elite bankers who rule the world's economics have a well-thought-out plan in full operation. It's been in the works for years, and we have been blindsided by their controlled media that tells us only what the elites want us to know. There is no such thing as freedom of the press. This Internet is well monitored, and hackers are working full-time to keep the truth in news off cyberspace. They knew very well they could enslave the world if they had total and unregulated ability to create unlimited wealth out of thin air – a world currency backed by nothing and accepted by the masses as trade for labor and real property. America is getting the slavery they deserved as they weren't diligent in protecting their God-given right to trade value for value. Can you imagine how those criminals are smugly enjoying the rape of our nation with inflation? They are having a heyday while our nation is literally going up in fire. They will make millions more on usury loans to those unfortunate folks that lost their homes to some degenerate arsonists.

It wouldn't be too farfetched to say that the same satanic forces who control our nation's wealth probably set the fires in California. You, the so-called intellectual-free Americans, surely know that if you allow a private group of thieves to offer their privately printed paper as your media of exchange and they retain the power to regulate the value of it, then you are the victims of the biggest fraud ever perpetuated on the human race. As the nation drives hell-bent into inflation and the dollar sinks into oblivion, the wealth has already been transferred into the hands of the elite. Land is the only real value left in our nation. Own it and get it out of the hands of the moneylenders. The Bible commands us to owe no man anything. Christians, get out of debt to the moneylenders. Governments, restore value and creditability to our dollar and back it with gold. They could never earn the right to own and rule our financial world as they have never put in a day's work in their lives. Parasites are bloodsuckers and do not generate value or earn status in the productive world of competition. Bankers don't compete in anything as they create their own wealth with an entry into their books. In the real world, they would have had to work, earn respect, and produce real value for their paper before we ever gave them that responsibility of regulating our world currencies. The so-called Federal Reserve System is not federal or answerable to anyone except the international entrepreneurs who are in control of all the world's resources. They are nothing but common criminals who do the dirty work for the bankers. They have divided the sheepling's groups like the Democrats or Republicans, white or black, foreign and domestic.

Clever means keep the world's populations focused on trivial things like a war here or there, a national fire or two, a good game of sports, and a constant flow of degenerate entertainment to rob our populations of original thinking for themselves. Television is the greatest mind-robbing conspiracy in the world. Television has captured the minds of our people and reduced them to a flock of pacified pleasure-seeking opportunists. You have no idea how well programmed and devoted the scriptwriters are in destroying the minds of our populations and our youth in particular. Have you been watching the garbage your kid's minds are being programmed with? This is a well-planned attack on dummying down the minds of our children. The cowboys and early settlers were our real heroes who built our nation. They established this great nation on godly values and moral values offered by Almighty God. Notice our founders brought the Bible with them as they pursued religious freedoms. As they settled in the West and brought prosperity to our nation and all its people, they exemplified true values and justice for all mankind. This new age movie junk using foul language, senseless killings, and sick sexual plots have all but destroyed the influences our forefathers had made on this nation. There are no more God-fearing heroes today in the media. It is all controlled by the atheistic globalists. I don't go to movies, nor do I watch the garbage on TV as I know it's geared to turn me into a mindless old man, discontented with everything God has created for me to enjoy. I try watching some of the preachers on TV, but they are always asking for money for some project that God cannot support. They holler as if God was bankrupted.

Spiritual men in tune with God will meet all their needs according to his riches in heaven. Man's natural desires should be confused with God's ministry for his creation. Our Bible stands on its own merits and speaks for itself. Preachers should be admonishing and encouraging their flocks. "If God be for you, who can be against you?" You see, it is easier to stir up the flocks by preaching platitudes and Bible stories than expose them to truths and facts that we are losing our nation to godless heathen who are driven by satanic forces to destroy God's creation.

Don't preach on the real issues facing our nation. Don't tell them we are fragmented into dominations and secular humanism. Don't preach unity and dedication to performing God's will on his earth. There is one God, one Jesus, and one body of believers on this earth. If pastors would quit preaching platitudes and individual interpretations, God could solidify the body of Christ on earth and restore peace to his land. You say that will never happen. Well, you're wrong as there is justice, heaven, hell, and God. You may never live long enough to see it happen, but when they start dropping a few well-placed atomic bombs in the world, you watch the restoration of the body of Christ becoming one voice again as in the old days. We all know that we are one in Christ, and it will probably take a world disaster to unite his body again as in the days of Paul of Tarsus. You know, I just might live long enough to see it happen. Globalists' greed is anxiety for power, and their lies will soon hit the fan. The people will get a rude awakening as the masses can no longer ignore their lying rhetoric. You won't hear division as the body of Christ will be restored with one bomb.

Our freedoms originate from God, which includes the freedom of choice that is offered by our Creator God. We Americans are very naive and trusting, and we are living in denial. We have given away our true freedoms to living in bondage to the destructive force of usury. Our nations and all their inhabitants no longer enjoy a free existence as their individual freedom and dignity are gone with the compromising of God-given sovereignty of self-rule. We have become a complacent population that is wrapped up in creature comforts ignorant to our addictions. Just put it on a credit card. We are living on the income from paycheck to paycheck while our nation is being rapped and plundered by globalists who treat all God's creation with contempt. They are using their media control as a tool for dumbing down the masses and keeping them in ignorance to the massive debt of the people. The world societies no longer encourage children to reach out to achieve their highest calling. They discourage freethinkers and want everyone to conform to the new age molds of accomplishment. Their programs of keeping the children ignorant are well in place; and only the few, well placed in special schools for the rich, can move up the ladder into full awareness. Every child is being promoted to think like everyone else and to believe that one system works for all. The present school system is archaic and geared to force everyone to conform to the so-called new age thinking. The human herd is being programmed into secular humanism and a microcontrolled thinking society. Everybody is being programmed into living in a herd, feeding at the bankers' troth, submerged in debt, working from dawn to sunset to make ends meet.

Leisure time is a detriment and threat to a controlled society. Spare time has to be programmed for the masses in useless entertainment to keep their minds active and focused on trivial entertainment. In that offering is the mindless TV talk shows and valueless, senseless movies that stimulate the imagination with sex, violence, dirty language, senseless plots, and excessive demeaning of our Christian values. Confusing and creating turmoil within our society is dividing our nation into being complacent and despondent to being a threat to the globalists' agenda. The mindless garbage on today's TV programs prevents the young minds from developing into mature thinkers as the new image glorifies money and sex symbols. The focus is on the pursuit of success and money, like *Dancing with the Stars*, *Deal or No Deal*, and *Who Wants to Be a Millionaire?* Notice that the focus of these games is on money. They are a big success as it stimulates the viewers with sexy women and charismatic announcers to stimulate the viewers. You see how the TV business is developing the mind-control shows that use entertainment as a form of brain processing that has the brain's imaginations running free with visions of success. This programming is directing your minds into living in complacency with false hope. They create a vision for the contestant that is unobtainable, and he then becomes a victim to his unobtainable wealth and greed that stays alive with hope. It's called something-for-nothing syndrome. The viewer loses desire and respect for himself as he is an unexpected victim. The person becomes depressed and not satisfied with his present condition. Life is a drag, a mundane existence settling for living in the herd of complacency.

Multiply that picture by millions of Americans glued to the TV tubes and you have the present nature of our society today. We sit back and watch the handful of greedy global dictators take over our government, our schools, and our churches; but what you really don't see is we really gave it to them. We have fallen prey to our own complacency being content with the subhuman standards of living in usury debt and enslaved by the desires of our hearts in material possessions. The herd has been given different levels of status within the society to give the humans a sense of being able to improve on their financial and social status in the herds. They are being programmed to accept their standard of living based on their contribution to the welfare of the elites. A powerful group of police have been set up as protectorates of the realm. The police state will give special perks to enjoy their status in the society, stabilizing their loyalty to the elites. Their primary duty is to keep the sheeplings in line and preventing a rebellion within the herd. They force obedience to their laws to govern the land and keep opportunities just out of reach. If they expect more out of life, then they are expendable for the good of all. The whole program is based on fear and is augmented with public entertainment that is based on what is good for the good of all. BS. New world standards will be set up for all people to live by; and if they become rebellious, then for the good of all, they are eliminated from the herd. When will the Christians stand up and claim this land for God and stop giving it to the globalists? When will they stop the genocide of the minds of all children? Where are the Martin Luther King, Jr.'s of our time?

Where are the great men who fought at Valley Forge for our real freedom? Slavery comes in many forms. When the mind and body are cluttered up with meaningless rhetoric, sick and loose values, and the object of affection is *money*, then the herd is in the pits. Is there any force left out there ready to stand up against the globalists' money and ready to restore sanity to our nation? Somebody needs to stand up and be counted for as our pastors are out feeding in the pastures. Our nation is going underfinancial with debt personnel slavery, and the pastors are holding retreats. The world populations are watching us as the masses are being enslaved into materialism, debt, and rampant crime that are all out of control. Our once-freethinking churchgoers are struggling and have fallen prey on usury, keeping up with the Joneses instead of seeking godly wisdom and direction to lead the force for God and restore our constitutional government. Don't they need to regroup by bringing the wrath of God down on the men who instigated 9/11 and bring them to justice? Preachers are blinded with regulations, preaching platitudes, prosperity, and Bible stories. Religion has replaced a dedicated service to our Lord's commandments. We prefer to be churchgoers and not responsible to God's commandments. We give lip service without commitment to his commandments.

Jesus paid the ultimate price to redeem our souls from a life of hell on this earth. He gave all mankind hope to satisfy his belief system, and he gave assurance for eternal life. I look back at my life and all that I tried to accomplish, and I realized it is but a waste without my faith and trust in Jesus. I have trusted Jesus for seventy-eight years, and he is best thing going,

Without my valid belief system, I would have to live my life by my animal instinct and write off any hope for life after death. Not a good deal as it doesn't solve the problem I have of being concern over death. Why in God's name can I imagine life eternal if it were not a possibility? If I wanted to gain everything I could for this life, then I would have been a banker or a politician. I would want to cram everything into this life as there is no hope beyond the grave. Do you not see why these bankers and politicians are so possessed with their material wealth and self-esteem? That's all the hope for this life they have to live with. Imagine gaining the world and losing your eternal soul. That price is too much to give for obtaining political status on this planet. I have no problem living within my means. When my last wife separated from me after thirty years of marriage, I thought my world had been devastated. I had heart problems and almost died. I was alone and had only God to turn to. God got my attention, and it was a blessing in disguise. I now have given a new bonding with a Christian wife who loves the Lord. We have a deep spiritual bond in Christ that has brought me enjoyment and deep purpose for my life. Marriage is not just living together having companionship. It is a bonding of two souls as one in Christ. It is a joy that passes all understanding as you are happy beyond your wildest dreams. It is a balance of emotions and contentment as you are never alone, and you put God into that scenario, and you have the perfect life. With the proper soul mate, there is no mountain you can't climb and no calling on your life from God you can't accomplish. I now enjoy the life God intended me to have while I live his planet.

Very few rich men enter the kingdom of God (Matt. 9:24). What can I say that will help you in making a commitment to "seek first the kingdom of God"? Is it asking too much to have you seek God's divine purpose for your life? Do you think for one minute God wants you spend your whole life seeking temporal material goodies? What a drag that would be! Do you expect him to add spiritual security on top of that with no real response from you? If you believe God loves you, then you also believe God wants you to return his love with your expression of love. What is it that is preventing you from accepting the real picture of the condition of our nation today? My assessment is you are not secured in God's love for you. Is it too late for our people to vote a change and restore sanity within our government? To force the leadership of the church, to hold fast to Christian principles, and to follow the Constitution and not the money? It seems there is a price on every vote in Congress. We need to vote in God-loving Christian men and women into our leadership; then we don't have to concern ourselves whether they are Republican or Democrat. They would hold loyalty to the Constitution only. Men and women who will stand up to confront the bankers' usury and restore creditability to our dollar (media of exchange), *gold*. Can we again learn to obey God's golden rule (Do unto to others as we would have others do unto us) and stamp out satanic usury that has bankrupted our people?

I have been given a prediction that we have a real wake-up call coming, and it is just down the street. Look for it. It's called 9/11 *upgrade*. This next one will make 9/11 look like a picnic.

The next criminal act of these world elites will cause a full-fledged collapse of our society, people starving with crime and panic filling the streets of our nation. There are three days' worth of food left on the shelves in the markets, and when that's gone, nothing else is in the offering. What? You called me a doom and glum spinmaster. Excuse me, it's not your back I'm looking after, it's mine and my family. The fact that I am verbal about the true condition of our nation and hope to restore sanity to the idiots who are perpetuating this train wreak is part of my nature. When I led the Arizona Patriots years ago, God first gave me the vision of the condition of our nation and its forthcoming bondage to world globalists' bankers. Why do you think the police came down on our organization so fast? Because we had some real radicals in the group who wanted to get armed and prepared to protect our Constitution from the printers of bogus money. I disbanded the group as I could see the confutation that was headed in our direction. It was not a win-win situation, and it may not be now. Timing is everything, and patriots are always at a disadvantage as the bankers have all the time they need to implement their agenda of world control. The Arizona Patriots were ready to take up arms and run the bankers and their stooges right out of our country. Most of them were ex-service men who had served in the no-win war of Korea and knew they were cannon fodder in the hands of the elites. The controlled stooges who run the church got irate and upset at my radical preaching and started calling me anti-Semitic and closed down my church operation. I am no more anti-Semitic than the pope is a Jew. The Jews are not at fault; in this matter, they are the victims.

It's the radical Zionists bankers who have taken cover under their banking institute and under disguise of being the Israelites. These Zionists are atheists who worship bale, power, and greed; and who pride themselves in being super intellects having put the Goya under bondage of their printed paper. They consider the rest of God's creation as sheep that need to be penned up and taught servitude to the world masters. They have grandeurs of dethroning God and taking over his world with the use of lies, wealth, panic, and fear. With the controlling of distribution of wealth and a carefully selective hiring of greedy personnel and politicians whose values are easily compromised with money, a small band of bankers have managed to take total control of the world. They used money and fear to buy the loyalties of government stooges. You see, government employees are a class of people who can't make it in the completive world, so they reduce themselves to parasites living off the productivity of the people and set up the bankers' protective services (military, Central Intelligence Agency [CIA], Food and Drug Administration [FDA], and the list goes on) and certainly add to that growing list the loyalty of most of our politicians. Their great fear is patriots, freedom-loving Christians, who will do battle against the criminals who want to take away their God-given freedoms. You see, they are willing to die for their great cause, and the bankers won't do that. They are smart and cowards as they get their highly paid stooges to die for them. Hopefully, you can see my wake-up call and take to task these treasonous bankers and take away their control of our currency.

Bring back the gold standard, stabilize our money, disband the Federal Reserve, and force our government to take on its responsibility of printing and regulating our currency.

Place all the leading banking counterfeiters in jail for life as they are a serious, evil threat to our constitutional republic, our nation survival, and our God-given freedoms. If they think they can get away with knocking down a couple of steel towers with preset demolition, killing our patriot presidents, bombing foreign nations for their oil, and controlling our brain-dead politicians who have committed treason against God's nation, brother, they have another thought coming as you can only push a Christian army so far; and God will raise them up to restore his *banner* on his chosen people. He will not give us up, and the American people are waking up; and someday soon, these subhumans will overstep their positions and get cocky and careless. The fires in California were purposely set, and it is my take it was a well-planned operation by an organization with a hidden agenda not considered by a trusting flock of sheep. Someday, truth will be revealed, and a Christian army will run these traitors out of God's nation and place them on to some remote island where they can devour each other. I don't doubt for one minute that they not are prepared for a revolt and an awakening to their treasonous acts. I'm sure, as our society starts to collapse into a dung heap, we will wake up; and I pray it won't be too late. My great concern is that they have control of the atomic bombs and would set one or two of them off to save their position of power in our world. Life has no value to them as they live without hope for eternity as their god is on earth, and he is a god that offers self-satisfaction in wealth and power. They live as fatalists without compassion and concern for God's creation. It takes a certain kind of degenerate man to create and use an atomic bomb on humanity.

They got away with it, bombing Japan, killing thousands after we were already winning that war. I can see a lot of you saying at this time, "Well, we saved a lot of lives." Have you ever heard of diplomacy? We could have just as easily dropped the bomb in some small island, and I'm sure they would have come to the surrender table. I feel the same way about taking over the world now for Christ. Need to force peace on the whole world even at gunpoint. I'm not so naive to think they wouldn't think twice about taking out a few million souls to obtain the world control they vision for themselves. They feel it as their responsibility to save the world for themselves as they are the elite thinkers who are more intelligent and can bring the world populations under controlled. They will stop contamination of the planet, control the resources, and create a perfect world for the few elites; and those who serve them are allowed to live. We are talking about complete autonomy with a police state where the rulers have complete control over life and death. How did I come by this knowledge and awareness? A lot of prayer and fasting, and I'm now on a program of fasting.

You can count on one thing for sure. Concern for God's created life on our planet is not their long suit. All life is expendable if it is in opposition to their agenda, and I'm sure they have paid assassins on their payrolls who are happy to do their dirty work. You see, when they print the wealth out of thin air, they can pay any price to have their sick agenda augmented. Pressure is building up for them as they see that the end is near; their propaganda machine of keeping the masses dummied down and uninformed is getting shaky.

The Internet offers free, up-to-date, and uncontrolled information going out to the people who want to get informed. The soon forthcoming poverty and shortage of food is something you need to be aware of and be prepared for as that for sure is on their agenda. Do you have any idea how easy it is to control a hungry population? We are a very instable nation; and fear is being used to condition the masses by setting of fires, blowing down buildings, staging wars for oil control, issuing constant barrage of health warnings, and instigating well-orchestrated brainwashing of the masses into a mode of pending fear and panic for a new savior who offers peace and security. Enter the new world order to bring hope and security to the masses who are still afloat after an extensive culling process. Our nation is sitting on the verge of bankruptcy, and the troops are getting restless. What kind of national disaster would it take to set our society into panic? It is fast becoming fragmented with no means of stabilizing itself, which makes it vulnerable to the new world saviors. Their army is a volunteer class of people who are living destitute, without hope or an education. The services offer some future and opportunity for a large part of our youth today. It is better they are put into the services where they can learn a trade and discipline. Also, they become loyal to the dictates of government and can be called up in case of a rebellion within the nation. The leadership are puppets schooled in the ROTC (Reserve Officers' Training Corps) or OCS (Officer Candidate School) ranks where they are taught to take orders without question or individual thought. I went through OCS and saw firsthand how we were being programmed to follow orders without question. Ours is not to question, just to do or die.

I fought their no-win, needless wars of culling populations and killing our patriotic young men. We are the best, most highly trained, and sophisticated armed forces on the planet today. Why do we need to threaten the world with atomic bombs and our powerful army? We have become the scourge of the planet as we now force all nations on our planet to prepare to defend themselves or give us all their natural resources and bow down to our power. No wonder we are the most hated nation in the world when we use to be loved and revered all over the world. Thanks, bankers. You have just signed our death warrant. Yes, there are nations who want us to be eliminated off the planet as we are a real threat to their existence. Yes, they are preparing to defend themselves, and they do have weapons of mass destruction. Greed is blind, but ego run amuck will destroy you off the face of the earth. We are the only real threat to life on this planet, and every nation knows it. You can be sure they are preparing to retaliate and wipe us of the face of the earth. Why are we not talking about getting rid of all weapons of mass destruction for the sake of human life on our planet? We all have equal right to live here. Yes.

The church is sound asleep (body of Christ) and living in fear of being closed down by the bankers as most of them are in debt to the bankers' usury. Shame on them. The world events presently unfolding should be considered by most evangelical believers as the unraveling of Bible prophecy as revealed by Bible scholars from the book of Revelations. The final tribulation could well be on its way.

The elite money changers who now control most of the world's resources, if not all, enjoy this biblical teaching.

It keeps the Christians at bay and in a tranquil state as believers enjoy taking a passive attitude that "God will sort out the mess we Christians allowed his planet to get into." They can dismiss any responsibility for the bankers stealing our Republic and putting our government and its people under trillions of dollars in debt. Many naive Christians overlook their treasonous actions as they can relate their actions to God's Word being fulfilled. That insulates them from having to be accountable and responsible for their actions. They just sit by and watch the destruction of our godly nation as it sinks into irreparable debt. How many times I have heard that it is prophecy just being fulfilled in our time. That is why these self-proclaimed world entrepreneurs are able to rapidly move ahead with their one-world government unopposed.

The continued wars between "useless eaters" are provoked and instigated by the bankers for culling of populations and perfecting a state of unrest and fear throughout the world. Our troops are being used as cannon fodder to perfect the agenda of the bankers of world domination. What an oxymoron; our military police actions worldwide is preserving freedoms and protecting our homeland from terrorists. A great lie as the opposite is true. Iraq War is an action for oil control and prevent that nation from dealing their oil with the Eurodollars for payment. It's about control of resources, and the gold of today is oil as they have confiscated most of the gold out of Fort Knox. The world runs on *oil*, and it sustains all lifestyles on our planet today with the use of oil. Some of the major reserves are in the hands of Arabs.

As an engineer working for Douglas Aircraft Company, along with hundreds of other engineers, I am fully aware that you can't physically knock down a steel building in its footprint with an airplane filled with gas. Heat generated from gas/petrol burning is not hot enough to melt steel all the way to the ground. Those building were preset with charges ready to be activated. They coordinated the demolition with the dummy airplanes. It's impossible to implode steel buildings without set charges. And there is no way you can knock down three steel buildings with two bombs. Bombed buildings don't drop straight down. Read "9/11was a Hoax" on the Internet. Get informed and learn the truth about 9/11, and you will be able to accept the rest of my ramblings. The elites are unopposed as they move our world under their debt system with usury and fear. The world trembles in fear of the consequences of compliancy and blindness as the silence is deafening. It's obvious they have the complete control of the press and our government puppets. They all are supporting the one-world dictatorship by their inaction and silence. The masses of this world have succumbed to fear, and the patriots/Christians have been silenced. The elites are culling the middle class out of existence as they offer the only threat to their world agenda of one-world government. The once-dominating middle class had been a thorn in their sides; however, that threat is silenced.

The prophecy of world tribulation is being revealed by many Bible scholars as the events that are now to take place on earth for the end-times of mankind's sojourn on our planet. As I said, the bankers love this prophecy as it offers them license to take control of the earth unopposed.

Prophecy Revisited

And there shall be signs in the sun, and in the moon, and in the stars; and upon the earth distress of nations, with perplexity; the sea and the waves roaring;

Men's hearts failing them for fear, and for looking after those things which are coming on the earth: for the powers of heaven shall be shaken.

— Luke 21:25-26

This know also, that in the last days perilous times shall come. For men shall be lovers of their own selves, covetous, boasters, proud, blasphemers, disobedient to parents, unthankful, unholy,

Without natural affection, trucebreakers, false accusers, incontinent, fierce, despisers of those that are good,

Traitors, heady, highminded, lovers of pleasures more that lover of God;

Having a form of godliness, but denying the power thereof: from such turn away.

— 2 Timothy 3:1-5

T HIS IS MY assessment of the condition of our world today. Give this some prayer and let me know if you're not in agreement or have any inspiration that you might have to add light to this important subject. Knowledge is power, and we need to acquire all we can get as the world is in a great deal of pain. Knowledge cannot reach a closed mind that's engulfed in his own mind-set.

Today, approximately 120 million American church members have very little understanding of Bible prophecy. Pastors are not teaching Bible prophecy because most of them do not like to address the doom and gloom messages in the Word of God that are related the present condition of our world today. If they were to preach on what is going on today in the world, it would relate directly to God's Holy Scriptures and they would have to close their church as the government system would come down on them like the wrath of God. They would all have to accept the wrath of the complete banking cartel as they let one get away with speaking the truth about our satanic usury system that has destroyed our nation. As things get worst and the great collapse of our nation is about to take place, maybe, just maybe, it will awaken the body of Christ and we will rise up the banner of our Lord and stop the insanity and holocaust that is about to happen. If the pastors were to unite behind God's Word and preach the gospel of the end-times, many God-fearing Christians might be spared from grief and destruction. They need to expose the truth about what is going on today. Do you think for one minute God would not bring a revival and restore our prosperity if we would throw the criminal bankers into the pits of hell where they would feel right at home? We would witness a revival never before witnessed in the human experience on earth. Men and woman would stand up to the bogus government tyranny and elect God's representatives, and the original constitution would again be restored as the law of the land.

Our people do not understand the importance of events tied in Israel and the Middle East nations.

They are not aware of the significance of the formation of the European Union. The world managers are so well disciplined and organized that the complacency of the world populations in accepting the one-world rulers is unopposed and well on its way to being augmented, if not already in place. Remember the forces of evil control all the media. They own the airwaves and have brainwashed the media to mimicking their agenda of world complacency and ignore the ton of evidence that is only available on the Internet. I call them the Fox News mummies who are being duped into being brain-dead mimics of Rush Limbaugh. He is an egomaniac who is nothing but a rich tool for the elite's agenda. They have silenced our prominent, constitutional, patriot newsmen by monitoring and crushing all descending truths with intimidation, money, and rhetoric of being non-American, not supporting our troops while ignoring and culling out undesirable patriots who have become victims of their proper gander.

They create their no-win wars of personal gain to cull out our patriot young men who could offer resistance to their agenda of world control. These young patriots represent the only real threat to their ambitions of one-world government. So they send them out to the foreign killing fields to fight and protect their personal interests in confiscation of all the world's natural resources. Vietnam War, Korean War, etc., are nothing more than propaganda wars of culling freedom of loving young men who believe America is the land and home of the brave and the free. They now have all but closed the door on our once-free society and have all their pawns in place to set up their one-world government.

Look at the Forces Of Evil

The international elites of world CEO bankers hidden in the Bilderberger Group, Trilateralists, and Counsel of Foreign Relations have successfully undermined the constitutional control of our Republic and are presently collapsing the U.S. economy into oblivion with servitude to national debt.

They have installed loyal members throughout government to run their one-world dictatorship. When a puppet politician sings out of tune with their personal agenda and tries to save or restore the Republic, he or she is quietly terminated like President Kennedy and many others. He is my hero, and he's a real patriot. I met him while we shot *PT 109* in Key West, Florida. President Kennedy tried to save our nation from the globalists by restoring the gold standard backing for the U.S. dollar. His presidential decree is still on the books. On June 4, 1963, Kennedy signed Executive Order 11110 that returned the power of the government to issue silver certificates against the silver bullion. All in all, Kennedy brought $4.3 billion in silver certificates into circulation. It would have prevented the national debt from reaching its present level as the government could pay its debt without going to the Fed Reserve criminals. Kennedy was murdered for his efforts to free Americans. Having a dollar backed by gold would stop inflation; Federal Reserve Notes (FRN), fiat money, couldn't be printed unless it had silver or gold in Fort Knox to back its value. We would not be in debt as we would be forced to live within our means. The gold standard would have restored our creditability worldwide, and we wouldn't be in debt to every nation in the world.

Only a token amount of gold is left at Fort Knox for people to see as it has been rapped and gold sent to Europe. Our nation is bankrupt, which is witnessed by our national debt ($8,995,850,677,373.96). Restoring gold is not an option as it was the law of the land set down by our founding fathers. The economy of our nation has gone to European banks, and our people with the nation are submerged in a mountain of irreparable debt. We are under in a big way as we spend $1.36 billion of debt every day. Folks, we are living in a borrowed time till that debt is recalled.

You now have a picture of your government's debt, and it still borrows money to support a war machine to enslave the world. That makes sense to you. Where are its priorities? What really is going on behind your backs that you are not informed about? You need to get mad as hell and start to harass your government to come clean. Why are they sending your kids to fight their no-win wars of debt to your nation and destroy any creditability you might have had in the world? We are the most despised and feared nation in the world because we have an out-of-control government, intimidating the world with our arsenal and destroying bombs. Have you heard about the new technology to kill humans? It's called antimatter weapons. The air force is spending millions to develop a radical power source – antimatter. It is the most powerful energy source known to man. It has been studied by physicists since the 1930s. Each subatomic particle has its antimatter counterpart. When they collide, they annihilate each other with a burst of energy that exceeds your imagination. It does not release radiation, but the heat emitted would fry any grid system.

However, that is not going to happen as this present society is focused on TV fantasies, money games, sex symbols, brainwashing of our children, and a mountain of sick entertainment geared to dummying down the minds of the world populations.

You see, if I told you the depth of true story of Hollywood's treasonous actions, it would put fear in your hearts and rock your security blanket to the core. For you to realize and accept the truth that a handful of mortal men could literally devastate our planet into a manageable herd with proper gander from Hollywood is not part of your mind-set. For me to prove that our nation is on a path of irreversible self-destruction could not be acceptable to the conditioned mind of complacent inhabitants living in denial on this shaky planet.

The fact that the world conspirators will continue to cull the world populations with wars, diseases, and toxic wastes is not on the frontal lobe of the minds of the masses. We are all focused on present events, sports, and pleasures with no awareness of the results of not being vigilant in guarding our constitutional, God-given freedoms. No one is addressing any of our problems, and our highly paid, insulated government is providing the mark of the beast.

To define the meaning of a capitalistic system of government is first defined by determining the meaning of *capital. Capital* is the physical possession of a known commodity (bombs, money, gold, oil, food, land, poisons, etc.) established as a vital resource necessary for sustaining man's existence.

A capitalistic government owes allegiance to capital, and the almighty dollar decides the course of action, not God.

By owning and controlling the gold resources of the world, the one-world conspirators, hidden in secret societies known as the Illuminates of Thanateros, Trilateralists, Bilderberger Group, Skull and Bones, Counsel of Foreign Relations, etc., have been able to micromanage the world. These world bankers have for years printed, owned, and distributed their bogus money as the only medium of exchange worldwide. These handful of international bankers have stolen most the gold out of Fort Knox and have moved it to secret locations in England. Read about "Fort Knox Gold." Gold has always been the stable commodity to give creditability to any currency that was redeemably backed by gold. By the use of usury loans, the international ministers have been able to place the nations in the world under usury debt, forcing them to compromise their sovereignty and succumb to the agenda of the moneylenders. Jesus threw them out of the temple, and we embrace them. We give them our allegiance and power of printing the almighty dollar to control the destiny of all mankind with their well-financed world governments. Take a little time and get informed as to what happened to your gold-backed dollar when they stole all the gold out of Fort Knox and moved it to Europe. In Internet page about "Fort Knox Gold," read it and weep. Get informed, people.

By taking physical control of all the necessary commodities to sustain life on our planet, the bankers' control of international commerce is now complete. Puppet governments worldwide have been victimized by power of the banking cartel of biblical money changers.

Governments have had to submit to the forced raping and pilfering of all their natural resources by having to accept in exchange for their real wealth – the bankers' counterfeit paper. The power to the printing presses and visual aids have offered the world bankers total control over international commerce. Governments will collapse in mass hysteria when the bankers' dollar collapses and massive starvation occurs worldwide. They own the guns, remember? Their plan is simple. All the societies of the world will then be forced into population reductions to survive in their world as there is only a limited resource of food available to feed the vast populations of the world. Let's look at a few statistics.

1. Every year, fifteen million children die of hunger.
2. In Asian, African, and Latin American, five hundred million live in poverty.
3. Three billion people struggle to survive on $2 a day.
4. Every 3.6 seconds, someone dies of hunger.
5. It is determined that eight hundred million people suffer from hunger and malnutrition. The assets of the world's three richest men are more than the combined GNP of the least three undeveloped countries on the planet.
6. For the price of one missile, a school full of hungry children could eat lunch for five years. What I see going on presently is a world

disaster that is purposely being ignored by the forces that could do something about it. If not soon addressed, it will bring on a world crisis that will change the face of our planet permanently. Where is the body of Christ today? Is it not concerned over the condition of our planet and its inhabitants? Is God not concerned over all his creation and the needless suffering that's going on in his world today?

Paper money is useless when food is not available that's needed to sustain life. The nation's leaderships will be forced to reduce populations into controlled numbers to live within boundaries of what the food source will support in the way of life. You see, the population explosion has started putting a strain on agriculture. As agricultural land becomes scarce and food production diminishes, governments will have to set a standard by which certain societies must downsize their populations. Nations who do not submit to the world's food-sharing program by controlling their populations will be eliminated from the earth by starvation. Sort of like the blacks in Africa suffering and dying from AIDS and food shortages. AIDS is a laboratory-developed disease. This means the elite brains of this world, our globalists, have set up programs to bring the world populations under control, starting with culling out the useless middle class who are educated, armed, and a real threat to their world ambitions. These useless eaters who do not serve the interest of the elites are targeted for destruction. They have education and affluence and possession of 200 million handguns. Thirty-three states allow patriots to carry canceled weapons. This group is not asleep as to what is going on in our nation and are starting to see clearly the planned destruction of our middle class. These common folks who fight their wars are starting to see a satanic agenda behind their no-win wars for culling undesirables, securing the world's oil production, and dominating the monetary system with worthless fiat paper. You see, Iraq made the mistake of wanting to move their currency into the Eurodollar, and Iran is making that same mistake.

Any sane man knows Iran is no threat to our nation or the world, just as Iraq had no weapons of mass destruction. They are nations unfortunate enough to be sitting on one of the world's largest oil reserves and wanted to disenfranchise themselves from our worthless dollar. It is amazing how most of the world can see the fraudulent value of our dollar is being dumped and are running to the euro as the international currency. Our masses only see what the globalists wanted them to see and read. It's our criminals in government who have compromised our laws that protect our society and that should be on the hook for the destruction of our society.

Our government has given the privately owned Federal Reserve System the total authority over the printing and distribution of our media of exchange. The bogus FRS allowed a handful of foreign aliens to print our money and place our nation's under financial enslavement to their usury uncontrolled debt system. These foreign bankers that stole our monetary system have placed every red-blooded American into their debt system for their entire lives. They have totally enslaved the greatest free society God had ever developed. The society has been reduced to the haves and have-nots. The whole fiasco of bringing down three steel buildings with two airplanes sucks! No pictures or parts of any airplanes have ever been found. They cleaned up the mess in the matter of days with dozens of workers being exposed to radioactive dust. Those buildings imploded in their tracks, and thousands of engineers like myself have determined that those buildings had been fixed with explosives. As I said, gasoline doesn't melt steel.

It doesn't take a rocket scientist to work that one out. Those buildings were brought down by traitors within our nation, period. To those brain-dead viewers who have bought the Fox News' doctrine, don't waste your time reading further as your minds have been programmed with a well-documented mind-control system that is a proven program of mind control. Your media has been programming your mind for years. We are all witnesses to one of the greatest atrocities ever committed against the human race. Mind control is the art of programming our minds in a manner that it believes and supports everything it has been programmed to accept. You will be voting against your own best interests if you vote for either one of presidential candidates that's being presented today.

What in God's name is going on? Why are we becoming victimized by our own system of government? Why would anyone in their right mind want to undermine our representative type of government? Well, the answer to that is very simple. If you have the evil desire to own and control a dying planet and the world populations, you must have an applicable plan to accomplish that feat. Bring fear and chaos; control the money, the government, the economy; and be ready to discredit the handful of patriots who are ready to stand up for the Republic. The masses, remember, are in a dreamworld, sound asleep. Certain freedoms are left in place to give an image of freedom to pacify those who are brain-dead. We are being led to believe we still have some God-given freedoms of speech and movement. We are still free to bear arms, and freedom of movement still exists. What is lost is the truth and exposure to the intents of the globalists.

How in God's name can you have freedom if the media is controlled and you are feed only with half-truths? The news is used to micromanage the populations who are keeping the massive herd of sheeplings still suckling on breast milk. Believing we are still living in utopia, centered in pursuit of life, liberty, and happiness. Wake up, Americans, church is out! The nation is under attack, and the enemy of personal freedoms and our God is about to perfect another world catastrophe that will make the 9/11 look like a picnic.

Distribution of all wealth is now in the control of the international bankers as the world populations are being micromanaged by their stooges. The culling of populations is presently being augmented as disease and genocide are out of control and wars are everywhere. All nations are being subjected to the new world order's agenda or starve from isolation and internal strife. They must accept the globalists' bankers' bogus currencies as their media of exchange. It is the people's fault their nation is in deep debt as our Lord told us not to get involved in usury. Jesus threw the money-changing parasites out of his church and into the streets. His only act of aggression recorded in the Word. What about the Bible verse to "owe no man anything." Usury is an abomination to God. Results are financial bondage, owing allegiance to your creditors, suffering from disobedience and the chastisement from God. Our nation has accepted bankers' usury as the norm as we all want what we can't afford. We all live on the income with a mountain of debt. You own nothing as you are living in your bankers' home, driving their cars, and paying homage to him every month by paying your usury bills.

Bite the bullet, folks, as we are a bankrupt nation, waiting on the bankers to close down the shop. We, the God's chosen nation to the world, are now reaping our disobedience to God's Word. This once-free nation of God-fearing souls has sold their nation to the almighty paper dollar. Those poor Arabs knew something we didn't. They wanted to exchange their oil for Eurodollars, a more stable currency. I wonder why. Could it be that those international bankers plan to use the euro as the world currency, and the dollar is being purposely dumped along with our nation? Check Bloomberg.com (Dollar approached record low against the euro after consumer confidence hits all-time low). So goes our dollar, so goes our national economy, and so goes your standard of life. If and when that happens, we all will lose value on everything we own. How easy it is to bring down a once great, stable nation who had gold to back up their currency. I wouldn't be surprised to see us all have to trade our bogus money in for an international currency as we are being forced into a one-world system. Iraq and Iran made big mistakes to think they could get away with trading their oil against the value of the euros. The U.S. oil barons were trading in U.S. dollars, and they wanted their oil to be marketed against their bogus dollar that they have total control over the printing presses. The only way they could secure creditability of their printing presses is to evaluate the dollar-against-the-oil demands worldwide. The Middle East oil producers wanted to be tied to the Eurodollar as it is the only currency in Europe whose value was set by the European globalists' bankers that is stable. The world is climbing out of the dollar as it is being taxed.

By switching to the euro, they would dethrone the dollar as the world's exchange currency and, at the same time, bring down American empire under the banner of the globalists' agenda for world control.

Iran has just made a move to trading its oil into the Eurodollars, and we are rattling our war machine against that action under the disguise that she is contemplating terrorism. Who owns the printing presses, controls the monopolized money that presently offers control over the economies of the world? The only means to stabilize the world's economy is to have a valid monetary system backed by gold. To assure the compliance of nations to their World Trade agreements, the elite bankers have stationed their highly trained police forces and U.S. military forces in over 140-plus nations throughout the world.

These governments have willfully accept their bribes – and the Eurodollars or international credit – to allow our forts and military personnel physical presents with total military movement throughout their nations. These forces are the visual protectors and intimidators for the globalists' agenda to receive unquestioned compliance to their one-world ambitions. The world governments are presently moving in to total compliance to the globalists' agenda. Only a few rogue nations are still holding sovereignty over their populations. They have bought and established army bases worldwide that are loaded with military and equipment, including atomic bombs for the purpose of intimidation and physical control over all earth's humanity. All nations are now aware that the American forces have the nuclear capabilities to annihilate their existence off the face of the planet.

The one-world degenerates are now set for the complete fulfillment of their world ambitions for one-world government. With their use of force and intimidation and no concern for God's creation, they could cause a devastating catastrophe to happen that will make 9/11 look like a picnic. These deranged souls are capable of doing anything necessary to fulfill their evil desires. Enforcing compliance to laws and regulations, they keep world resources and profits flowing in their direction. Check "America's Empire of Bases" that enforces their world corporate control of the entire world. The world corporate managers are also about micromanaging all life-sustaining commodities needed for sustaining human life on this planet.

They have methodically maneuvered the puppet governments of the world into accepting their power and prestige into becoming their guardians, protectorates, and dictators. Every international business structure is being controlled by the new globalist currency, Eurodollars. Most of the world societies have already become totally dependent upon the internationalists and their bogus paper money for international trade. The bankers have most of the world in debt to their bogus money. Every penny you borrow is created out of thin air and placed on your grave as debt to the world bankers who never worked a day in their lives to earn your hard-earned labor. You are enslaved into their debt system that robs you of your work, your hope, and your future. As long as they can develop debt out of thin air, all societies are doomed into financial slavery.

In order to continue having the victims accept private paper notes, they devaluate their paper in exchange for your goods and services.

If I pay less for your labor than the inflation rate of eggs, you are led to believe you are getting less compensated for your labor. Wrong, as it is the value of your paper note that is going down, not the cost of the eggs you're buying. Your dollar is buying less is what you're led to believe when in truth, your price of food is going up faster than your dollar value. Your boss is stealing from you as your labor worth is being dumped against the food you need to sustain your life. Ask yourself, has your groceries bill gone up? If so, why? Is food source scarce? Is the farmer cleaning up, or does inflation affect him as well? Since the dollar has no stable value and it is no longer attached to the value of gold, then it's valued at the mercy of its printer, the globalists' bankers. That, folks, is Catch 22 and a license to rob their victims of their hard labors. While you're making the same money, it's being devalued as the price of commodities are going through the ceiling. While everything is going up, the value of your dollars is being dumped. Just look at the price of gold. It is going through the ceiling, and your dollars should be right with it. Do you see why the globalists' FDR system took away your gold and placed you into perpetual struggle for financial security? It's all about control and reducing the middle class into financial slavery by struggling to keep their heads above water. It's a process of slow drowning so you get used to living without hope. It's a well-thought-out program, and it will work as the people are pacifist and want to live a tranquil life in the Republic that their forefathers left them. Their media will not indoctrinate the masses as there would be a rebellion overnight, and bankers and politicians would go to the gallows.

That will never happen as the globalists now have a well-trained police force on their payroll that are living high off the hog. Patriots are being channeled into the armed forces where they are cannon fodder for their beliefs that we are fighting for a noble cause. Since when was stealing gas and oil from weaker nations not a noble cause? Folks, be objective and realize that there are no accidents, and everything has meaning and purpose behind the action. There is no threat from any nation on this planet against our superior armed forces. People do not commit suicide for a lost cause, even if they are Arabs. Two or three well-placed atomic bombs and the whole nation goes up in a cloud of nuclear waste. Let's get real, folks, wars are about ideologies and material gains. In the case of our globalists, it's all about world control, starting with America, the beautiful. They have the biggest gun on the block, and so they deserve to run the world. The problem I have with that is we are turning our world over to a group of evil, satanic worshipers who hold no respect for God and his creation. They will destroy our world just to fulfill their inflated egos. The globalists are now prepared to live underground for the rest of their lives to accomplish their evil goals. Their bogus dollar is the greatest scam ever perpetuated against the human race. Their paper is worthless; the whole world knows the bankers are bankrupting the human race into a world of debt. The only way you can stabilize the world economy is by restoring the gold standard as the only medium of exchange. All goods should be evaluated against the value of gold, and that value can be determined by its need and creditability in the human market. In any case, you are trading your labor for equal value.

The world has become intertwined economically; thus, nations are becoming dependent on each other. A prime example is when Venezuela government stops its oil production, the price of gas is affected worldwide. All social structures have become totally dependent on oil, along with other key products, forcing governments to conform to the agenda set by the one-world managers – who have prevented other energy sources from being developed.

Do you realize how easy it is for those in control to develop a world famine or energy crisis? Take this for example, create an urgent news, release it like "this is going to be one of the worst flu seasons in decades." Then follow that with a statement from the pharmaceuticals that there is going to be a shortage of the flu shots. Expose a few people getting sick and dying on media outlets – presto, you're out of product and billions richer, and the problem goes away. Notice today that nothing more has been written about a flu epidemic. My readers, that is capitalism at its best. It feeds of fear and ignorance of the brain-dead masses who support everything they read as they have no reliable access to truth in media except a few Internet Web pages. There are a many bogglers who offer readers unbiased truth in world events. Jeff Rense and YouTube offer a constant valid analysis of the truth in journalism as the capitalist news system has become greedy and has sold out their integrity to the almighty dollar. There has been for years an uncontrolled ravishing and raping of all news resources worldwide. The use of the media is to control, cull, and enslave the world's naive populations.

The moral foundations in the world has been raped and demeaned with God's awareness isolated out of public exposure and offered only in the church. The masses have lost their confidence in their ability to tell right from wrong. They prefer following a charismatic leaders who will do their speaking for them. These so-called spiritual leaders are dormant or brain-dead in the Revelation from the Bible that clearly depicts our world facing the end-time prophecies as clearly offered in God's Word. The church is dormant, resting in the comforts of a healthy congregation, readily meeting their financial needs. How can they ignore the signs of the end-time? How many homes, jobs, and lifestyles must be lost before they wake up and start to evoke God's will into being prepared for the end-times ahead? The pastors are optimistic as they are dealing with the symptoms and ignoring the cause. No one like doom and gloom, but how long do we have to suffer before someone brings out the truth of what is presently going on in our nation? It doesn't matter whether you're a Democrat or Republican, all heads are being programmed into moral materialism that has become the official religion of the world's public societies. Read Stormfront.org. Television has become the biggest merchandiser of a false sense of security and confidence in our government's integrity.

The human herds are programmed to feel that they are in control of their governments with their vote. That's a lie straight from hell. Bush stole the last election with his judges, and we all knew it and did nothing to prevent it. Those programs – like free elections, free movement, free speech, etc. – offers the world herds a false sense of freedom. Hogwash.

It pacifies the skeptics and keeps the herd living with a glimpse of hope, fear, and creature comforts from within the confines of their holding pens. Ninety percent of families in the world live from paycheck to paycheck. Ten percent of the world's population control 90 percent of all wealth. Anyone who tries to expose or disrupt the world manager's agenda for world domination is quickly rejected as extremists and anti-Semitic or silenced.

Read mwhodges.home.att.net. Zero tolerance for dissentients. All that is demanded is enjoying a world of lemmings traveling along a narrow highway, conforming to their hidden agenda of war-peace mind-set. While the subjects are preoccupied with subliminal affairs of state, they are being systematically herded into a one-world society of subhuman existence. With the use of trumped-up world terror, prolonged fear, and financial despotism, they have all the herds confined into holding pens. Freedom is only a mind-set and belief system propagated within a media-controlled lifestyle. Ignorance is bliss, and what you don't know or have knowledge of you will never miss. The Internet is the last bastion of free speech, and it is fading fast. You are only being allowed to see a small part of the real picture. Prime example is the pharmaceutical advertisements as they spew out their propaganda, "Have you asked your doctor about the purple pill Nexium?" Then they go on into a spiel about the advantages of using their drugs, follow it by a short discourse on the side effects that protects them from personal libel suits. Your death from the use of the drug has no effect on their sales as it will not seem be newsworthy in most medias. Certain bloggers have come to the rescue like Jeff Rense.

Death at the hands of the pharmaceutical drugs that doesn't make profitable reading as it angers one of the medias' strongest clients. It's all about greedy capitalism. When the doctor says it's okay, it has to be okay, and he has the complete support of the entire medical cartel behind him. The worst scenario he faces is a personal lawsuit for malpractice. Doctors are the third largest cause of deaths in our nation because of faulty misdiagnosis of treatments. What good is it to collect a large settlement when you're not here to enjoy it?

How could this ever happen to a so-called free and open society. Well, it all really started in 1903 when the Congress of our Republic committed high treason. Article 1 section 8 of the Constitution says that only Congress can have the power to create money and regulate the value thereof. They gave up that coveted responsibility to a handful of international private bankers now called the Federal Reserve. Look up "Federal Reserve Fraud" on the Net and get informed. Read it and weep as you will see the greatest treason ever perpetuated against the human race. Our founding fathers knew well how important it was to maintain and control the coining of money to sustain a free society. Read week13-golbalization-moneyfraud. I like expressing some of this treasonous act in my own words; however, there are other patriots out there who have devoted their life to protecting our freedoms. Financial institutions are now preparing to collapse our capitalistic societies into total oblivion and set up their new world order. Fort Knox's gold is now in sitting safely in Bern, Switzerland, in the hands of the globalists. What is really going on with this world's power play?

It looks as if our nation is the prime target for spearheading the total control of all mankind. Well, there is no known means to control man's greed and desires to be like the Most High. We were a nation governed by Christian ethics. Christian concepts taught in his Word – render to Caesar, turn the other cheek, do unto others, love your enemies, etc. – were predominate influences in our society. That mind-set has been undermined and confined to being taught in most churches. Is there a positive solution to this coming destruction of our freedoms? Yes, but I am sure you're not prepared to make that sacrifice, not at this period in time. So I am going to leave that discourse to the last part of this book. Besides, it is only my opinion that I have interpreted from the Bible's prophecy and other profound spiritual ideas. I can say this, however, maintaining your health plays a major part in your ability to survive the forthcoming world collapse. My last thought on this matter is God has not forsaken his chosen ones, and when the fullness of his time has come, he will intercede into the affairs of mankind. That is a fact of life as our creator will lead and bring justice into his creation.

Now look, let's have a look at this same picture from the manager's side of the coin. The world managers are satanic, secular humanists who worship the superficial power and money that were afforded them in this corporate world. They live a hopeless, feudal existence and are the most insecure group of inhabitants of the human race presently existing on our planet. They meet in secret forums and in far-out, secured surroundings with no exposure to the world. They have bodyguards and constant surveillance of all the people around them.

They have to live with constant sense of fear of their lives from the free people who value their freedom and are fearless because of their faith in the living God. These globalists are constantly having to monitor the world populations just to assure themselves that everything is going according to their evil plans. They are so possessed with their agenda to control the world that they have become blindly entrapped by their obsession for world power and blatantly unconcerned over the welfare of the masses. They harbor total contempt for all God's creation as they have an agendum that is infallible. They are starting to celebrate as the Israelis did on that roof, watching the towers that totally collapsed. They are rejoicing as they have enslaved the entire world to their worthless paper notes, the Federal Reserve Note. They never entertain embracing real values for life as they have no belief system that answers to a creator. I wonder how they think life started and keeps going without a force if they can't see it doesn't exist. Truth is not a reality. They will die in a state of denial, depression, and solitude living a miserable existence, possessed by fear and inner emptiness that come with being a multibillionaire. The saddest part of the picture is that mankind has always had to confront these elite secret societies, greedily seeking control of all mankind with fear, mind control, money, and power. Our history is filled with their senseless wars of greed from the beginning of recorded time. History seems to always repeat itself as greed and insecurity follow man everywhere he goes. His uncontrolled desires plague his life to the grave. His inner need to find divine meaning to his life is a driving force to deal with.

His subconscious mind seeks contentment and peace for his soul within. Every obstacle we face has some meaning and purpose for life that we choose to ignore. This is the natural condition of natural man without a born-again experience with his Creator God. His soul is living his life separated from the love and comfort from his Creator God.

The most important mandate the globalists were able to instigate into human politics is separation of church and state. They prevented unity of God's laws and the divine-proven principles of those laws benefiting humanity through government. They took God out of making decisions for our nation and replaced him with the root of all evil – love of money. The reason they used, I'm sure, is the bickering and belittling over Christian doctrines, terminologies, and divine meaning to God's Word. Instead of coming together on common ground and fighting the common foe of secular humanism, they removed God from the process and left their government in the hands of the greedy moneylenders. It is easy to see that the globalists were successful in keeping our nation divided and vulnerable to the interest of the globalists. We are reaping pure hell from the division of the churches, and our nation will not survive until we bury our biblical differences to bring unity to the body of Christ. The church leaders prefer to live divided, priding themselves in being supporters of their unique, the only correct, interpretation of God's Holy Scriptures. This leaves the body of Christ divided and doomed to every whim of secular humanistic doctrine that creates an atmosphere that Jesus purposely divided his flocks so they could be picked off by the wolves of Satan.

We are doomed for destruction as a Republic as we are presently witnessing the failures of a secular humanistic government whose leaders offer their votes to the highest bidder. You might say the Bible enforces the separation of church and state, but you are wrong. Our present satanic government has no interest in enforcing church policies and principles as it cannot adhere to its teachings of "love your enemies, turn the other cheek, pray for them who mistreat you, don't fear for tomorrow, and lay your treasures up in heaven." I'm sure you are aware that the secular churches are equally guilty as they do not address the issues in state that opposes God's laws or the protections of human rights as demanded in God's Holy Scriptures. The churches would lose their privileges and be reprimanded with losing their tax-free status. What is more important are our freedom and right to hold God up as the principal founder of our Republic in our schools, church emblems in our public places, and government role in maintaining this godly endowed nation who follows after God in all his decisions. That, my dear readers, has been squash and only a remnant is left of the church's influences over our government. The state has silenced the God of our nation and taken control of the affairs of mankind, leaving the church with a small window of influence in reaching its souls for God. The state is a satanic tool now used to divide the body of Christ on earth.

As species, we are on the brink of a passage into a new form of living or existing on this planet. The old ways has been discarded and deemed archaic and unproductive. We are no longer a Republic.

We have no way of knowing if a true republic could achieve a greater degree of justice for mankind because no actual republic has ever been left totally in place as it gave too much freedom to the individual who always produced a tyrant that abuses his freedom. The old European systems produced endless wars and toxic graveyards throughout Europe. This leaves us to wonder if a true democratic republic would even work if implemented correctly. Humans are unable to resist material corruption: everyone has a price beyond which their morality fails. We have, by and large, abandoned the exhortations of Jesus to love our neighbors in favor of the bogus belief that money can immunize us from morality. The choices are clear; it's either tyranny or enlightenment. If the bankers don't merge with the churches and develop a universal currency based on morality, fairness to all humanity, and the mutual welfare of all the world's inhabitants – it will sink into oblivion. Governments must protect the survival, comfort, hopes, and life of the present human experience; or it will collapse in a dung heap, if it hasn't already. Capitalism has failed because it relies on slums in which to dump its failed products as well as an unregulated fluidity at the top with which to constantly bail them out of their overly greedy ventures. Socialist systems have never succeeded to overcome the privilege, authority, and tyrannical corruption that evolve out of noble intentions for the masses.

No government system ever devised a method on this planet to place the control of its natural world resources, which belongs to the world's community, into the hands of all its inhabitants. Corruption has always prevailed, and it remains uncontrolled.

The elected manage to make off with the loot, leaving the true owners of all God's natural resources high and dry. This is how our religions and governments have failed us as the earth's natural wealth belongs to all its inhabitants. Mankind cannot obtain true freedom as long as the money supply is in the hands of the few elite and usury is the means for mankind to support his life. The religions of the world have failed the mankind as they have not thrown the money changers out of the church. We can never aspire to a higher awareness as long as we are enslaved by usury. We will be forced to live in a controlled society of the haves and the have-nots. This leaves mankind living in fear of being one bomb away from having in this land blessed with fire. The task of attaching a moral quotient to money may be an impossibility as it would place a limit on man's freedom of choice so another approach must be considered. The real underlying problem in the world is the practice of usury by the international bankers. Usury is voluntary slavery, and an immature, uninformed society will run after temporal goodies and not concern themselves over the bondage they now live under. Usury allows the bankers to privately lend or print wealth, but they hold autonomy over the borrower. They also can determine who can obtain that wealth and who can't. By selectively determining who can have credit and who cannot, they can put the wealth of the world into the hands of the few who agree with their political philosophy. If you oppose their world agenda, then your company just might find itself bankrupted as your competitor has access to unlimited funds. That's how the rich got richer and the poor got poorer.

That's how the wealth of this world is consecrated into the hands of a selected few. You have heard the saying, "You have to have money to make money." Our Western civilization has been built entirely on usury. What good is the massive, modern skyscrapers that express the excellence of our civilization when they are monuments to greed and power that serve to prove that usury is the means to build an empire. The rest of the people on earth are there to serve the elite moneylenders and offer services to run their profitable businesses. Could it be that one day we evolve to a higher awareness of God and are willing to trade our skyscrapers and our usury bondage for an altruistic system that produces happy, self-reliant communities, living within modest means and virtues? The megalopolis are impressive from a distance because you can't see the bodies of the homeless moldering and dying in its windswept alleyways. As long as money power is in the hands of the few elite rulers, the world inhabitants cannot truly rule themselves. If we are not ruled by godly virtues, then *we will be ruled by tyrants.*

The godly man who evolves to a higher awareness is seldom heard by the earthlings as his path in life takes the high road who seeks no worldly recognition or personal gain. His affections are focused on service to all mankind, and the fulfillment of his God-given created purpose for his life. That is not the accumulation of temporal goodies that perishes with the holder. The elite, unfortunately, are not able to live in love, peace, and harmony with their fellow man as they are endowed without of control-inflated egos that are driven with a blind assumption that they are like the highest God.

They live with no loyalty or principles outside their greedy self-desires to control all the earth's resources and inhabitants. They don't belong to the natural human race as you and I know it. They, by their own choosing, live as a separate species on earth, whose existence is terminated upon death. History records over and over again that that form of humanoids, living possessed with their power and self-expression, are doomed to self-destruction. I'm convinced at times that that species of mankind was not created from any godly force. That humanoid form exists with no visible concern for the mutual welfare of human existence on this planet. These are the kinds of animal forms that create and develop weapons of mass destruction, new man-eating microbugs released in public, and famines that destroy millions. How can any sane, loving, caring human born of a woman dedicate his life and all his given talents developing the means to control, destroy, and annihilate his fellow man? *The New Nuclear Danger* by Dr. Helen Caldicott, a pediatrician dealing with babies and their growing disease problems with a nuclear-contaminated earth, has done extensive research into the new developments of nuclear bombs being developed by our government. You must get this book as not only it will convince you to look after your own health, but it just might motivate you to get active in the plight of man's ability to survive a nuclear holocaust being developed right here in the good old U.S. of A. I want to review a small part of her book which was well documented. National Ignition Facility (NIF) at Lawrence Livermore National Laboratory in California is presently developing or has developed 192 separate laser beams.

The energy released in bursts of three billionth of a second to a level of 1.8 million joules of energy. This will reach a temperature of one hundred million degrees centigrade. This condition only exists in the center of the sun. When this work is completed, it will produce a pure fusion bomb, which would be undetectable by a satellite. For your information, plutonium named after Pluto, the god of hell, remains radioactive and biologically dangerous for five hundred thousand years. It is the most carcinogenic substance known to human beings. It is said that one pound, if evenly distributed, could induce lung cancer in every person on earth (*The New Nuclear Danger*). What would it take for some drunken idiot with his hand on the switch to desire to see what that button will really do to mankind? Just curious bystanders, or I call them look-y-loos. Hope you will read her book.

Well, one thing for sure, the world is changing fast; and many governments in our world today have the means to destroy all life on this planet with one, single push of a button. Now, doesn't that excite you? What a great leap of accomplishment for mankind! I just wonder how our Creator is going to deal with that one. I'm sure he is not pleased with the indiscriminate, dirty bombs now being dropped on his creation in Iraq. Skylax@comcast.net – this is also a must read as it is better stated and documented.

Foreign government's political leaders are underwritten by the world managers to enact laws to protect their capitalistic marketplace. They have set up their low-cost manufacturing in these countries with very little obstruction from their highly paid government cronies.

I lived in Costa Rica and watched Intel Corporation put up a factory across from my place to produce microchips. They were able to produce those chips for pennies, paying cheap labor and without retirement benefits to their slave laborers. A prime example of just how the megacorporations are rapping all the world's resources while destroying their economies by keeping the masses poor. Our government passed a new law that Bush signed on prescription drugs for the seniors. The media tells you that it will save the seniors millions in revenue. Hogwash. Some will benefit, but who is the real, beneficial heirs? Big corporations who had offered their workers retirement drug benefits will now enjoy having the government pay for those prescriptions with your tax money, saving the pharmaceuticals millions each year. I don't blame the world managers as they are born into their situation in life and know no other calling. Our politicians are the prostitutes and criminals as they have sworn to uphold our Constitution that protects the rulers of this nation. The present group of spineless wonders will not rock the boat that keeps their goodies flowing. There is just one or maybe two statesmen left in Congress. One is Congressman Ron Paul (projectfreedom.com). He is a real Texan and statesman, not a cowboy who says, "Bring 'em on" as thousands of souls are murdered for oil. Ron Paul deserves to be president of our Republic, but I doubt he would live long enough to enjoy to see our nation return to constitutional government.

All natural foreign-owned products, vital to man's survival on earth, are subject to rape from the world bankers. Their products are controlled with their bogus international currencies.

Those third world nations are not allowed the use of a currency that has any international value, so the World Bank is able to float that nation's economy with debt to the globalists' interests. Colón of Costa Rica was a hundred and fifty to a dollar when I was there; and it is now, three years later, at 419.68 colónes to the dollar. Their money isn't worth the paper; it's printed on outside of the nation. The political prostitutes who sell out their countries to the bankers keep their bloody money in offshore numbered accounts just like the megacorporations. You don't think they are going to pay taxes, do you?

The world managers, in order to maintain the total financial control over all third world nations, pick their leadership, school them in our colleges, and support their rise to power in their countries. These young and ambitious kids are schooled in the capitalistic system of debt, money control, and have embraced the new world order for total population control. They have bought the elites' agenda of what is good for the world management. You see, the dialogue is the same. The world is overpopulated and needs management. The higher privileged elite must step in and take control of resources and population explosions before the world self-destructs. You see, having wealth gives them a sense of superiority and privilege. It doesn't make any difference how they made it or what they use it for as money brings a sense of power and independence. They take it upon themselves to save the world from destruction. A noble jester accepts they are the self-proclaimed rulers and they will determine who lives and dies. The elites are going to save the world for themselves.

You see, I believe that action is necessary, but not from the viewpoint that human life is not sacred to God. You can't treat life as it is a commodity. You must have respect for all life as it belongs to its Creator God. My approach in dealing with the population explosion is humanitarian respect for God's law of "thou shall not kill."

First, you need to expose and educate the world to the real condition of our planet. The saturation of mankind will create a toxic famine on earth where thousands will die of starvation disease. The major pollution of the world is with the toxic waste of mankind.

Our earth is designed to support a certain amount of life, and we need to determine that number and move toward holding the world populations to that point. We also have to consider God's animal creatures in that analysis and make ample space for all of them. We'll need representatives from all nations in working together to gather and document that information. Our one-world humanity survival committee will gather all the information vital to make this happen and bring it into all the nations for final approval and ratification. We need to get the best brains in our societies to serve on this committee. Also, set up an information-gathering center to have the whole world populations involved in offering input to the committee. In-depth educational program is vitally needed, and greatest brains on our planet should be involved. We need every nation to embrace the concept and agree to support the final, overall plan. This, dear friends, is the sane way to control the assured disaster this world is facing. We need to combine the use of our experience and technical knowledge to find the means to live in peace.

We need to stop immediately the building of weapons of mass destruction and destroy the arsenals that exist. Also, include other weapons now being developed to destroy God's creation. The superpowers could make this happen and demand universal support to "save the planet." We are aware that many endangered species are now losing numbers and many have already become extinct. This has to stop, and we must embrace an alterative method to preserve all life on our planet. Greed and power must step down, and inspiration from God must prevail.

The world leaders and intellects need to come together and devise a plan to save the planet, not destroy it to a toxic waste field. We need to save it from ourselves. The taxpayers have been bled out and can no longer carry the cost of government's agenda for world control. Excessive spending wastes especially when the government spends more than it collects from its herd. As you're aware by now, corporations don't pay taxes; they just pass that cost down to the consumers. We are facing a well-planned collapse of our once-free society as we slowly descend into a capitalist-controlled depression. Our once-free nation is now facing the need for a new peaceful revolution to restore our constitutional form of government. I leave you with my one great hope: there is a God who can intercede and answer the prayers of his believers. I believe that is the only hope for mankind at this present time in history. This ongoing spiritual war is between powers and principalities. The prize at stake is the very souls of all mankind. If the present-world, money-printing elites win this war, mankind will face the total devastation of God's planet.

Free, God-fearing men will never accept the slavery that has been planned for mankind on this planet. There is no way in hell you can take away mankind's hope for an eternal place with his Creator. If you think for one minute, Mr. World Elites, that you are going to get God's creation and believers to lay down and live in slavery due to the use of fear, you got another thinking coming. We, the believers in Christ, are void of fear of dying and live with hope and security that our lives have conformed to principles laid out by God. Lost souls and minds have chosen to live separated from a belief system in God.

Pleasure and self-edification is their escape from the reality that their souls are lost and going to hell. Without a valid belief system in God, they live off temporal enjoyment and derive security in money as it gives them self-esteem in the insecure, materialistic world they live in. You live in total fear of the unknown as you have no belief system to secure life after death. In short, live without hope being wrapped up in flat money notes that become the object of your affections. Now that you see my overall picture of our world's condition under the rule of usury capitalism, then you can understand why I feel so strongly that your health is being programmed into that scenario. One of the agenda of the world managers is a well-planned program of culling the world's populations. Unprovoked wars, starvation, unaffordable health care, and a total financial disaster is the well-conceived condition of our world today. Our elite masters plan on accomplishing that feat by no-win wars, releasing laboratory-grown viruses and controlling the medical system, toxic contamination of selected societies, and on the near horizon, World War III.

By allowing their manmade diseases to run rampant throughout the world societies, they think they can generally cull the populations into a controllable numbers while at the same time rapping millions in medical services from the victims. Health services are just another capitalistic controlling device. Maintaining good health by exercising your free and obtaining knowledge will prevent your life earnings from being confiscated by the clever manipulations of the medical cartel. The health care industry consists of the medical profession, insurance industry, pharmaceutical industry, hospital industry, and the banking conglomerate. These are trillion-dollar capitalist systems exercising total control over the health industry and the health of the world. If you are still one of the gullible souls who think a few Arab terrorists are the primary threat to our so-called free society, then you should open your eyes to the medical cartel controlling your health and well-being. With its present strangling halt on all government's medical policies, they will be slowly negating your right to have access to natural, alternative means for curing yourself. You cannot fully understand the magnitude of this injustice of negating your access to alternative cures until you are faced with a debilitating disease where you have been told to go home and die. The system has given up on you as you are probably broke and have nothing to offer to the system. You are left to seek out other means to sustain your life. Cancer victims are prime examples of patients with little or no know-how of alternatives for affording a cure for their disease. Did you know that there presently exist many natural means of the curing of cancer that has been squashed and defamed by the medical cartel?

All that wealth of information is being discredited or suppressed by the capitalists as it is a major threat to the well-established, highly creditable cancer research system that has been researching for a cure forever.

One must realize that one cancer patient cured is not only the loss of capital but a setting of a very bad precedent for millions of potential victims. Now, I hope you can see that your life is a commodity and you are being treated by the medical cartel as a cannon fodder in the open market. You're just another dollar figure to enter in the profit-and-loss statement. If you think for one minute that your life has more importance than that to the medical moguls, then you're living in denial and dreamworld that could cost you your life. You get cancer, and the last place you want to go is to a cancer doctor. Nature paths have a far better record without burning your guts up with radiation. Corporation America just sent our freedom-loving soldiers to fight in no-win war for the interests of a handful of oil barons and bankers. Energy resources are the greatest control force in this modern world, and the force that controls that depleting resource controls the destiny of the human race. That struggle for energy control will not go away in our lifetime as it is the commodity that maintains and sustains human existence on this planet. Culling the world populations is not an option but a necessity for the world managers. Government controllers have now determined that human life is an expendable commodity (collateral damage). They are using their nonending planned wars of sacrificing surplus humanity to achieve their imperialistic agenda. God has promised in his Word not to intervene in the human affairs until the last days.

That day might be coming alone sooner than we think. In the meantime, I believe the most important issue facing your present existence is to acquire faith and love of God with his wisdom on how to keep your life on this planet effective, strong, and free from all diseases. The battle for your freedoms is within the powers and principalities of this world. Your move is to live to be a part of his plan for mankind on his earth and to be prepared to be divinely called in these trying days. This book is dedicated toward bringing you to enlightened information so you won't miss that calling. Read it with one thing in mind: to get well and stay well and pray for the gift of love and true compassion for this suffering world. That's all the depressive political garbage that I am going to share as the rest of the drama is being played out daily in your media. You want to keep up with the world events, go to rense. com, and get all the bad news on daily basis. I might warn you that it is somewhat depressing to read the truth when you have to sit back and turn loose and let God.

Preface Two

NOW LET US focus on a few simple, health-sustaining facts on how it is possible for us to live in this polluted society with optimum health. Keeping an optimistic viewpoint and enjoying continual health without the threat of the medical care systems raping your children out of their inheritance. We are going to explore hundreds of sharing of God-loving people who are willing to reveal their findings and studies on natural cures that they have documented and have proven to be effective in obtaining and sustaining optimum health.

These dedicated souls have found the means to express their findings on the cyber world and books, which is a creditable task as they are being harassed and persecuted constantly by the controlling freaks of the medical system. Capitalism is highly motivated and dedicated to destroying any or all opportunities you might have of curing yourself through natural means.

The procurement of having and maintaining good health in today's society is a serious game as you must now be aware that the deck is fully stacked against you. Along with the capitalists' medical monopoly, there are thousands of opportunists and witch doctors hard at work out there, pitching for your last will and testament. The present government-supported medical cartel has purposely separated our society from knowledge, past and present, on how to keep our lives naturally running at optimum condition. "An ounce of prevention is worth a pound of cure" is a lost phrase. We now live in the new world of media mind control, promoting "a pill a day keeps the doctor away." The pharmaceuticals have replaced the wisdom of time and proven natural remedies of our forefathers with the quick fix and the miracle pill. Cures from God's natural resources found throughout the world have been abandoned, discredited, or purposely hidden by the medical cartel to protect the wealth of the medical capitalists.

Cures that are found in nature cannot be patented or monopolized by the megacorporations; therefore, they cannot be tolerated to exist in competition with their capitalistic system of total control of all the world medical services.

We may be living longer due to an easier and more comfortable lifestyle.

Who did that survey? The pharmaceuticals. But we certainly are not living healthier lives. The tremendous pressure of teenage crimes, drugs, illiteracy, homelessness, financial problems, and over 50 percent divorce rates is just a few things that bear witness to the ongoing devastation of our once-God-inspired free society. Can you imagine how far along our natural health techniques would be if we were implementing some of the modern technologies, directing money from half of what we spend on weapons to improving our knowledge and applications of known natural remedies and cures that have been passed down for centuries from our parents? The medical system has totally depressed our God-given rights to that natural, historical health cures that had served our needs for thousands of years. We don't see doctors making house calls anymore as they are too busy trying to pay for their malpractice insurance. Something has to be done to revive sanity to our medical system. Doctors are being limited and intimidated by rules and regulations set by government regulating institutions. They can make no claims and give no assurance of cures for anything. They are schooled to diagnose and prescribe drugs as treatments for disease and must rely on the pharmaceutical companies' drug analysis for the effectiveness of their treatments. Their tests take years of blind studies and megabucks to perform on a selected group of guinea pigs. Wonder what percentage of success they have to have before they can get an FDA approval? I do know that the druggist come out with a bunch of restrictions and warnings directed at the users in the form of a list of reactions that might happen if used improperly.

It's simple it if you die from overdose tough luck. I think I would rather put my health into the hands of a Zulu medicine man in South Africa. I saw them perform some weird things, and nobody died.

The natural health industry has really only two effective means of support for their cures. One is the personal testimonies from the naturopaths who have documented the methods, amounts, and cures that the treatments have perfected. Second is the documented effects and responses to the personal care and effects as recorded by the patients from the various natural treatments. If those natural treatments directed at the whole body electric, had no effect, did no good, then you would never hear about it from anyone. People, don't get excited about failures and certainly don't pass misinformation and failures down through the test of time. Books, Internet, homeopaths, and naturopaths are the only avenues left open to patients seeking natural health remedies. Unfortunately, when it comes to your personal health, it is not likely that sufferers from chronic disease will put a lot of credence to unfamiliar natural remedies and the testimonies of strangers. Without *doctor* in front of their name, we are programmed to believe that there is no creditability to the remedies. The use of natural substances doesn't seem to fit into our fast-moving lifestyles. We require the quick fix, and a doctor who has gone through rigorous education and training to become licensed and certified to *practice* medicine. The hidden agenda behind this program is that more than half of them are incompetent and are in it for the money and prestige. Maybe that's why our doctors are the third largest cause of deaths in our country.

These deaths are all accidental, of course, that's why doctors have to carry the highest forms of medical insurance. They are not getting much help from their fellow capitalists, are they? You know, I would chose to die naturally in my sleep or on a bucking horse, but certainly not to be just another statistic on an insurance claim. Collecting that claim is not going to do me much good when I'm not around to enjoy it.

One of our God-given inalienable rights and responsibilities is to choose for ourselves how we desire to take care of our own body. The treatments we determine to use must be our own choice, and not made from a medical system run by the pharmaceuticals. Therefore, it should be mandatory that every patient have access to all information, knowledge, methods, and options available that deal with their health situations. Doctors should be required to tell patients all their alternatives for treating their illnesses. Tell me, why isn't my government allowing that information to be exposed and revealed by doctors? Why are natural cures that are proven effective from years of use not being certified by the medical system? Why am I being kept from using natural products such as Laetrile, colloidal silver, magnetic pulsar, Zapper, and many other methods proven to be effective cures for disease? Why isn't our government looking after the welfare of its rulers or subjects? Shouldn't natural remedies be documented and proven with blind studies and medical supervision the same as drugs? The proven creditability and benefits of all natural remedies that have been around for centuries should be made to be part and parcel of our choices for all medical treatment.

Just because they can't be patented shouldn't be the determining factor to me by not having access to cures to preserve my life. All medical options for me to obtain a cure (synthetic and natural) should be laid out on the table by my doctor for me to choose and determine for myself.

My grandmother gave me god-awful-tasting homemade slurp that cured my strip throat every time within three days. I have no idea what was in that stuff except the blackstrap molasses, but it worked better than any drug on the market today, and I don't know how to make it as she has gone home to be with our Lord.

The closed society of today's modern medicine is so well protected by the pharmaceuticals and government that it has imprisoned the minds and lives of the masses. It has entrapped the loyalty and servitude of the sick and the dying, leaving them with no other creditable alternatives. Their medical victims who never realize that the medical system never offers a cure for anything, just a treatment, a temporary fix while the body, if it can, is forced to cure itself. Perfecting cures for disease would put their industry out of business and develop total chaos for a multibillon-dollar capitalistic gang of thugs who relies on your blind loyalty for their existence. This ignorance is magnified and supported by the public, soliciting of donations for so-called nonprofit organizations. These tax-free donations are directed to finding cures for cancer, AIDS, diabetes, and hundreds of other known death-producing diseases plaguing our society today. They serve two purposes. One, you are reminded that there is no known cure for your illness; and second, it maintains creditability to the system as it shows good faith.

They will perform and find that miracle cure someday, if you live long enough. What it really does is to discredit all other methods of curing your diseases, thus demeaning the natural health industry of homeopathic cures. We have in the meantime hundreds of other incurable, newly discovered diseases popping up in our terror-indoctrinated society all the time. The disease business has run out of names, so they are now using letter words like SARS, AIDS, CDN, mad cow, and now the bird flu. My guess is that they will have a bunch of new ones emerging before I can get the book out to press. What are your chances now of living out your normal life expectancy with optimum health? To my knowledge, no one has ever run a poll to determine that factor as that is probably information that the pharmaceuticals would not like to be publicized.

We Are What We Eat

L IVING IN A *corporate-controlled capitalism*, synthetically structured chemical food is the main source of food being offered to the herds to sustain their lives on this planet. Just as drug cartel creates pills, drugs for temporal pain relief that dampens the cries of "please help me" while the body reeks with pain. The fast-food cartel or our synthetic food industry is producing substance to only pacify the body's need for substance to fill the gut and offer some nourishment. Now, what exactly does this really mean to your life? It means that your body cannot sustain your health living off a depleted, undernourished, synthetic food supplements.

It also means that if it doesn't have the resources and vitality to give your life the energy it needs, it will deteriorate, and a disease will terminate its life on this planet. If you are serious about curing your body, then you must start eating natural foods that offer minerals and vitamins that are needed to support all your body's natural functions. The body was created to react to natural elements for its survival. This book makes no apologies for the truths that disrupt your complacent lifestyle, and I am just one caring, concerned soul who has witnessed the loss both of parents to medical cancer industry at a very early age. I stood by helplessly and watched them die a miserable, painful deaths while the medical system stripped them of all there dignity and earthly possessions. They gladly given up all their worldly possession just for one more day of life. My grandfather, Daddy Dewey, lived to be ninety-four; and Honey, my redhead grandmother, died in her sleep, dreaming of going home to be with God. She was a real pistol and gave me the jest for life that I have in God. She carried me off to church every Sunday – come rain or snow. I'm sure she is giving God a run for his money somewhere. I have left the comfort and security of being in tune with the will of God many times, but my indoctrination as a child within the body of Christ has brought me back to the fold and given me comfort in my times of self-involvement and out-of-control, egocentric living.

This experience with death of my parents was so close to home that it has made a lasting impression on my life. I have been purposely retired from the brainwashing film industry for twenty years.

I just didn't fit into the new Hollywood agenda of sex, violence, and child-mind control. Now living in full bloom at seventy-eight, I am on my way to recreating perfect health in my life so that I can witness to others, firsthand, the astronomical changes that are taking place in my life and on this planet. The enjoyment of living to see other citizens obtain knowledge and valid natural cures found on open markets is on my front burner. Without going through the gory details of my many worldly experiences, good and bad, up and down, I am now focused and determined to dedicate these last wonderful productive years of my life on God's earth to enjoy people, seeking truth and putting maximum effort in getting this book out and into the hands of my receptive fans. If I could just help one person enjoy a longer and disease-free existence, as Clint would say, *that would make my day.*

My primary goal is to document and expose all the pertinent information that will allow you to protect and produce a healthy, vibrant life to enjoy a full and rich life span in a contaminated world about you.

embrace these proven concepts. I will continue to spend all my spare time researching books, Internet, nature paths, newsletters, and whatever other sources of reliable information needed to put this book into the class of reliable and pertinent life-giving knowledge. The truth will *set you free*. I will continue to add to this information as buyers will also have the option of being put on my e-mail and newsletter's list for upgrades and new discoveries and exchanging information and testimonies. I have nothing to sell but knowledge and experience, and that I freely give.

There are hundreds of documented alternative methods of assisting God in the healing and maintaining the health of your neglected body. Life or death is not just a throw of the dice. The life you had been given did not happen by accident, neither will your death unless you are run over by a Mack Truck. We can become the authors and the finishers of our personal health. The Internet, applied with common sense, has exposed a wealth of health information that has offered a few of us inquisitive, self-motivated, common folks an opportunity of a lifetime. We can seek, study, test, and find extensive, reliable support knowledge and other information of the free world of electronic treatments to diseases. We can tap into an unlimited source of knowledge from all parts of the world. There are exhaustible, experienced, God-loving, altruistic men and women out there in cyberspace who have dedicated themselves to informing, documenting, and sharing testimonies of hundreds of natural, healthy experiences in healing the body. These common laymen, with a godly commitment to natural life, are helping hundreds, if not thousands, of people like yourself find a perfect, normal, healthy, long, and productive lives. Sure you'll find that there are crackpots and charlatans among them who are trying to convince you to buy their proven snake oils, but should that stop you from seeking and determining the truths on health practices that may cure and preserve the life that belongs to you? Laymen with no medical backgrounds have been dedicated to giving us inspired, well-documented, proven, natural health cures from personal research and remedies passed down from generations before them.

They are doing what your parents no longer have time to do. These home cures may very well be inexpensive health supplements and programs that have been well documented through the test of time. Some of these ancient methods are able to cure any and all forms of malfunctions and sicknesses that our bodies can come up with. A world of knowledge and confusion is open to all for the taking, and I have only begun to touch on exposing the mass amount of that information offered in this book. It would take volumes to process all the information available. I would remind you that I focus on where you can find the information and highlight some of that information for you to investigate for yourself. It will be up to your instincts and common sense to research the fullness of all the information and knowledge that's offered in this book.

I have been down to many dead-end roads and blind alleys in my endeavors to seek the truth on health cures. Nothing good ever came easy, thus the years of dedication and tenacity to bring forth the truths I have found for myself to share with you. I'm not here to sell you anything except to share access to the experience and knowledge that I have acquired over the last ten years of my life. I would like to help you reach a ripe old age of disease-free living. I don't pull any punches, and I tell it just as I have learned it – the hard way. You may resent accepting all of what I have to say, but I'm not running for president. I'm dedicated to the presentation of facts as I see them. Methods, that if applied as documented, have been proven to work for hundreds of victims of this polluted planet. You have all been brainwashed by media saturation that is money oriented.

You will need to make a strong commitment to seek the truth for preserving your health. Truth and only the truth will help you to overcome the powerful forces out there, dedicated to taking your last buck just before they put you away in a pine box. This is not a pretty picture, but life's a bitch, and then you die. Take control of your life now.

I have found that most of what we experience with any health program given by doctors and naturopaths supporting natural cures is trial and error as every person's body functions and metabolism are unique. No one fits all molds. Just look at our DNAs as a prime example of the unique creation of the human race. So with that simple statement in mind and having given you a truthful look at my intentions with this book, let's examine a positive direction of keeping and maintaining a healthy existence of a polluted planet. Remember, this book is designed as a stepping-stone, a reference point, for you to take control of your own health practices. My deep incentive for practicing what I preach is that I intend to leave all my earthly treasures to my kids, not to a flawed medical system. So join with me in this endeavor in obtaining all the knowledge and understanding necessary to develop a personal program for sustaining your God-given right to a healthy, rich, enjoyable, prosperous, and long life. It is going to be an exciting venture as the world is drastically changing right before our eyes, and I won't be there when God steps in and deals with this mass insanity that's going on around us. You can't enjoy the world events if you're struggling daily to keep your body alive. I credit my present optimum health and desire to help others to God's natural cures. God's wonderful, caring souls are my real heroes in this book. Their work and dedication to revealing natural health cures to the world is now noted and praised by this grateful and humbled admirer. I will be referring and relating to their tireless work throughout this book. Dr. Hulda Clark is one of those saints I want to talk about, and how she is being attacked by the whole forces of the medical managers. She is a seventy-six-year-old Mennonite who is sending the CEOs of the Pharma Cartel into seizures with her various books: *The Cure for All Diseases, The Cure for All Cancers, The Cure for Advanced Cancers,* and *The Cure for HIV and AIDS.* These books can still be purchased at your local health food store, and thousands have been sold, and millions more should be sold as they have helped and cured hundreds with the self-help approach that she advocates in her books (declare.net). Another saint who lives on the edge, giving the drug pushers and toxic waste distributors a run for their money, is Kevin Trudeau, whose books are on the New York's bestseller list. He is truly a modern-day whistle-blower who deserves the distinguished service medal for his contribution to mankind's inalienable right to proof and knowledge of the garbage they are eating to preserve life on this planet.

I also sincerely believe that we are all godly created individuals, possessing a spiritual awareness who gives us abilities for insight and confirmation to those methods and processes that serve to support and enhance the natural functions of our bodies. In a nutshell, we can know from our God-given instincts what is good for us and what is junk when we feed our bodies from the corporate troth.

People like to say that truth is different for every person because each body has different conditions, and I concur as truth in the health field industry has to be determined by individual needs that he or she faces. Truth in the health field is what natural treatments works for my body that restores and maintains its optimum health. I evaluate health information through extensive study and testimonies from creditable sources that have nothing to gain except blessings from God. That method of research and information that I have collected over the years are labeled and documented in this book. This is not an exhaustive study as it would take volumes to cover all the remedies used by various cultures throughout the world. We are going to focus on just a few programs that have been tried and proven by myself and other close associates. My attitude and actions directed toward sustaining my optimum health is simply defined as this: *if you can catch it, you can get rid of it.* No one I know has abused, misused, and defiled their life and body more vigorously and stupidly than *yours truly.* I have stumbled and crashed through the mainstream of Hollywood's crackpots for over forty years, I have been there and done that in most every adventure one can travel in over forty nations on this planet. I have, during that forty-plus years of playacting with over hundred films and TV shows under my belt, collected good revenues for playing the self-evolved egomaniac who showed absolutely no respect for his own personal life and limb. I have totally ignored the natural laws of cause and effect. I was a basket case awaiting cremation when God's eternal love intervened in my life.

I had been run over by a stagecoach, bucked off many a horse and bull, clobbered by a stuntman, had my neck broken by playing football, shot, drugged, beaten up by irate boyfriends and stuntmen, and am now living with a steel knee, a broken neck, and a separated shoulder – just to name a few of the many disorders and ailments brought on by my self-afflicted, aggressive, masochistic attitude toward life. Apart from the few aches and pains, I am in perfect health, enjoying a full range of exercises and sports.

Disease is running rampant throughout the world, and it is a trillion-dollar business out of control, so we need to address that as well. Apart from my little arthritis, my health is in optimum condition because I do all the right things. It took me seventy-odd years to learn the importance of taking care of my body and its health needs. I hope you're not one those pessimists who believes we can't cure some diseases when we can go to the moon, Mars, and wipe out all mankind in a few hours. Cures for all diseases have been known to exist for years, but these cures are suppressed by world managers who have no intention of disturbing the billion-dollar synthetic drug industry. Medical profession worldwide has grown into the second largest population-controlling profession known to modern man. The first being our globalists with their highly compensated politicians who are enjoying the politics and intrigues of global warfare. These barbarians, with their money power, are enjoying the world power struggle that will go to any ends to protect its stronghold on the populations of this world. The culling of the world populations is supported by all governments whose politicians are on their payrolls.

It is never the intentions of that cartel to cure disease as it is not profitable and does not fit into their overall plan of reducing the world populations.

I have attention deficit/hypertension disorder (ADHD), and I have had it since my erratic early childhood. I am now dedicated to controlling that known disease. I am presently turning my life around from an aimless world wanderer and an impulsive hairbrained decision maker to a spiritual-driven man, seeking daily God's purpose for my existence. This book prayerfully will be the evidence of my dedication to the perfecting of a cure for my life. Every ounce of self-discipline I can muster, along with my wife's loving support and patience, is going into defeating this disease naturally. To create, develop, and market this book as meaningful expression of love and concern for my fellow fans and readers is on top burner of my life – and truly a full-time task for me. You who have supported me in my first life have given me the incentive to work long hours and late nights just to make a clear and precise presentation of this second life. The forty-odd years I spent dedicated to bringing entertainment into the world will be totally lost for me if I can't turn that exposure into presenting something beneficiary and productive for my fellow world inhabitants. I have witnessed lately many of my close actor friends dying of various diseases without being given much hope from the medical profession. Disease is running rampant in our society with no control in sight. So let's tackle the issues that will offer a lasting, disease-free existence along with a purposeful existence with your Creator God. All things are possible with God.

By all rights, I should have been deceased years ago as with so many of my contemporaries who have moved on. Living in the fast lane in the Hollywood's environment, one may suffer from many illnesses, likely be run over by a stagecoach, wiped out in a stunt gig, or shot by a cowboy who forgot to load a blank. Hollywood life is very demanding as I did most of my own stunts and all my fight scenes. It seems we are playing some kind of role from morning to night. The only escape from fame is sleep and drugs. It warps your mind and molds your lifestyle into perverted sense of self-importance that after a while become very boring and robs you of your real person. So I am writing on borrowed time and will finish this book only with the help and mercy of the living God and my last wife and soul mate, Carolyn, who has been beneficial in restoring and redirecting what is left of my life.

Most of the material on natural healers and naturopaths, I have examined for myself and can testify firsthand to their declarations, expertise, experiences, and creditability on the natural cures for human health. They are not part of the multibillion-dollar synthetic health care industry that is notorious for killing more people than it cures. Trick statement as the body cures itself with our help or hindrance. This industry continues to grow, and new methods and cure-alls are being developed daily as the big pharmaceutical industry needs new diseases to keep its massive industry strong and prosperous. An example is AIDS, a bioterrorism infection that kills twice as many blacks, Latinos, and Native Americans than it does with whites.

The products of the natural health industry are so vastly distributed among many small-to-large companies in comparison to the pharmaceutical drug pushers, which has its consecrated money and power held by a few trillion-dollar corporations that maintain a stronghold on most the medical profession. The scenario used by many natural health companies is to assure their clients that they have the complete line of the best health products on the market; however, most of their supplements are made by four or five major manufacturers. Many supplements have additives that are fillers and toxic to sustain shelf life. Because they say it's natural doesn't mean it is not toxic. Cyanide is natural. Many natural supplements are no different than the synthesized drugs your doctors have you addicted to for life. We are going to address all these issues as I think it is important to get pure products that contain the vital supplements that enhance our life functions, not tax our immune systems with more toxins. We live in an imperfect world that's motivated by money, not the saving of lives. We have to deal with imperfection with tenacity and a positive attitude, looking for positive results.

I am now convinced that one cannot focus on just one aspect of your health without dealing with the whole body electric. Most doctors are being trained to treat systems of health problems as offered by patients or determine the extent of illness through tests and examinations. You can only relate to knowledge that have been taught and acquired in the medical schools. Have you ever had a doctor who gives you the known cause of your problems like you're eating wrong foods, not exercising properly, having too much stress, not taking enough sleep, etc.?

Doctors can only treat the systems that they have been schooled to recognize the cause of the problems. Cures are not part of the process as that is left up to the body. They put cancer in arrest for a period with slash-and-burn tactics of chemotherapy, which is noted for killing everything that is good and bad. What about the patient dealing with the cause? Only a few natural health practitioners have been schooled to address the major causes of cancer as that is a well-keep secret.

There is no pretense of me being a natural wellness guru or having any complete knowledge on any given health problem. Natural health procedures offered here are expressed in a manner that everyone can easily digest and determine if the information is applicable to your life.

I make no claims other than what natural cures has done for me. You will have to become your own doctor and make your own decisions on health supplements you take. One thing for sure, they will be all natural and will have very little or no side effects. Knowledge, along with experience in natural cures, is power that can make a difference in curing everyone's life as it gives the body the opportunity it needs to cure itself. Millions of people over the years have enjoyed and testified to beneficial cures from all sorts of diseases through the natural practices expressed and documented in this book. The material in this book is public domain and covers all sorts of human ailments from cancer to memory loss. Nothing in your life should carry more importance to you than your personal health. You don't have to be on your deathbed to be aware of how important enjoying natural cures contributes to a fulfilling enjoyable life.

If you can read this book with an open and receptive heart, you will know that this retired actor who gave the best in front of the screen and stage is offering the very best health information and practices that are available from the world of cyberspace and the natural health practitioners.

I am not only a firm believer in God's unconditional love toward mankind but practice daily the projection of unconditional love toward all my fellow inhabitants on this planet. I believe that this is the major key factor to a peaceful coexistence with all God's creation on this planet and a vital key ingredient in sustaining natural health. Wars for greed, power, and prestige are expressions of mass insanity and sickness that presently possess the minds and lives of our globalists' rulers. We are faced with the reality of the existence of weapons of mass destruction in the hands of these globalists' tyrants who are capable of terminating all life on our planet. We need to express agape love to our fellow man and awaken ourselves to the present insane agenda and practices of the world managers. With the unceasing threat of continuous wars of greed and power along with the massive medical industry, human life is truly in peril. The underlying message in this book is to propagate and express my deep conviction that the only action that can save our present, modern world from self-destruction is for mankind universally to develop and express unconditional love for all God-created organisms. "As we sow so shall we reap." I can offer you nothing more healing than for you to have access to lifesaving information that would propagate peace within and without.

Healing is a process of the body healing itself with natural support from herbs and foods that become an expression of God's love in you and for you. My efforts to this end is to encourage my readers to the awareness of how they can personally maintain their health in a hostile environment. This is accomplished by having total inner peace with God and a knowledge of his natural cures with his herbs and supplements that will perfect a cure in his body that is in tune with his God-given right to optimum health.

This book is designed to inspire you to seek deeper knowledge of your body's needs and functions. To know the methods of treating your body to the natural aids it needs to cure itself of any and all disease. To use your own natural instincts to seek health and happiness for your life by introducing you to the world of God's natural cures that were designed by God to keep you alive and kicking on his planet. To help you assume personal and total control over your own life and health. I have experienced and proven this program for myself as well as many others whom I have learned these from. I haven't been to a doctor myself for ages except to get my prostrate reamed out. Maintaining my health is also a constant, daily dedication to my spiritual wellness as well as the physical. You cannot divide your physical life from its spiritual identity. My personal observation is that we have to exercise a balance in our lives with the choices that we make for ourselves. We are body, soul, and spirit; and one cannot perfect a cure on one without addressing the needs of the other. We deal with our spiritual life because of the known effects of stress, anxiety, and grief put on our physical health through illness.

To cure the body and leave the mind and soul stressed out and in turmoil is a great injustice to our health. Sickness will remain a threat until the soul is at peace within the body. So much of your life experiences with good health is grounded and rooted in having a peaceful existence within your soul that assures you that all things are working together for your good. You must develop the unwavering belief in your ability to exercise self-discipline and good common sense necessary for obtaining and maintaining optimum health. All this can be obtained through a genuine belief in God as Creator. God can take on many expressions in this life, but one thing must be in common. He is your Creator and the focus of your spiritual love and affection. Without his help, you can easily fall back into the old established patterns of self-pity and envy. Each morning, we must renew our inner commitments to self-preservation and coexistence with God before we get up out of the bed. Don't think for one minute that we can exist on this planet without the sustaining power and the infinite love of your omnipotent Creator God. Remember that the acquired habits of living a debilitating and destructive lifestyle have been in total control of your life, mind, and egos for years. Awareness of the importance of living God within, maintaining and working with me and for me in sustaining my personal health was the furthest thought in my life. I didn't see that God had a part in this program until I had a out-of-body experience facing death. That vivid experience seeing my lifeless body stretched out on the floor of my apartment, totaled out with drugs and booze, convinced me that I had better seek God because my life was in the pits of hell.

You see, at that point in my life, I was on a self-destruction path toward hopeless oblivion. I had done everything, been everywhere – and life had no excitement or purpose. There was always a pill, a bottle, or some drugs to suppress the symptoms of body-and-mind deterioration. I had confidence that my body's immune system would remedy any problems I might have with health. I just didn't realize that I had reached the end of my body's ability to save my existence on this planet. My life force was depleted, and I was living off borrowed time. Well, that's water under the bridge. Hopefully, you are younger than I am and can start altering your lifestyle to overcome the pitfalls of a degenerate, brain-dead, and complacent lifestyle void of God's influence. Accepting God as a vital part of this equation while working out your own salvation with fear and reverence is and the only solution you can rely on for full recovery.

Through a focused meditation or quiet time every morning – renewing your commitments to change your health practices with the daily exercise of living, with the desire to accomplish your self-made goals for a healthy living – you will slowly experience spiritual and physical health healing along with a deep desire to serve our Lord. I don't care how ill you have allowed yourself to become, but you can get well and stay well. Life will take on a positive vision of mental healing, and that will bring on physical and spiritual abundant life. With your mind and action focused on a purposeful direction toward your daily activities that previously might have been just a mundane existence, you will restore vitality into your life and spirit. This scenario has worked wonders in my life and hundreds of other souls.

I now challenge you to give your life a self-imposed, positive healing and meditation, an opportunity to work within your life. My meditation or quiet time focuses every morning just as I get up to face the new day. I do not allow my attentions and thoughts to be diverted by focusing on the mundane, normal tasks of surviving the day. It starts with my being grateful for all God's expressions of love around me and for another day on top of earth. I am fortunate in living in the country that still has some freedoms with freedom of locomotion. I have God's beauty around my home with green trees and vegetation all around our house. The realization of his unconditional love toward me is expressed in all his creations, and expressions of love are sprayed all around our home. Every morning I just have to stop, focus on my life, and totally become aware of his expression of life all around me in the birds, fish, squirrels, chipmunks, rabbits, my wife, and family, to name a few. I am seeking today to live in harmony with my God, environment, and all the creatures that coexist with me on this planet. This includes the ultimate creature mankind himself. (There is no need to struggle to be free; the absence of struggle is in itself a freedom.) Trumgpa.

Within this book, you will find chronicles of what I and hundreds of other souls deemed to be the most vital and valid health information available from all over the world. This is not meant to be an exercise in literary eloquence but a simple synopsis of basic, pertinent information for any curious souls to understand, learn, and apply to one's personal life. This book decrees that you alone should have to take responsibility and control of your mind, body, and health.

It's been my experience that if you focus your energy, persistence, and perseverance to any health issue in your life, you can and will succeed in overcoming that problem and your self-esteem will reward your life with dividends beyond your wildest dreams. That physical change won't come overnight as our faulty conditions took years to develop, but the mental focus and assurance of success can begin now. We started developing cancer in our bodies years before it becomes prevalent. We should now make the decision to take control over our personal health before the body becomes so run-down and beaten up that it is a major struggle to survive daily. We should not wait until our bodies are so pained, reddened, and parasite-infested that they dampen our desires and drives to obtain and maintain optimum health. My grandfather always taught me that "an ounce of prevention is worth a pound of cure." My grandfather lived to be ninety-three and died in his sleep, dreaming of bass fishing, with me steering the boat for him.

All the sources of information enclosed have all been researched, practiced, and documented by me. I have personally gathered and condensed this information for your evaluation and application. You can go directly to my sources for broader and deeper understanding from those I consider vital contributors, whose lives are dedicated to revealing nature's great methods for self-healing. This book is not copy-written and protected by any law. You are free to distribute and print it at your discretion. I make no claims of healing power and have no natural products to sell, nor am I declaring or prescribing any miracle treatments. This is a testimony of all the methods and basic treatments I presently use.

I have researched, witnessed in others, and documented to place in this book for you to analyze for your own benefit. The health path outlined in this book is no cakewalk, and I work diligently every day at keeping my health at optimum performance. The older I get, the harder the program becomes, and that challenge stimulates me to become more and more dedicated and determined in my goal to live a disease-free life. I work in my garden, play golf, work out regularly, use the computer, take saunas, and meditate (pray) on a regular schedule. I am very careful what I feed this previously abused old body and now concentrate on eating at least 80 percent of my food living (fruit and vegetables). Healthy living is a difficult, demanding task in this present environment of fast foods and manufactured dead substance being passed off as nutritional food. We are devout social creatures and are accustomed to eating what is being offered to us at social functions. Our money-orientated media discredits or ignores health freaks who live of raw foods, and we get very little exposure to the fast-food moguls. As a new health freak, I have no status in this immense culinary society of fast foods and corporate-controlled management of the food supply. This book will not be in the top-ten best sellers. As the selected few that will read this labor of love, I strongly suggest that you manage to hear me out as you may never hear this message again. I understand there is a bill before Congress to outlaw natural supplements and vitamins and put every form of health aids under the management of the FDA. That will cause the natural health freaks to have to go underground. This is a serious problem as Mexico and Canada are where we would get supplements and herbs.

This proven program for optimum health will require you first to change your mind-set on what is determined to be food for your life. This might require you to make a total lifestyle change. In most cases, it will take the ultimate sacrifice in altering old established eating habits. Many of you will not find the intestinal fortitude (willpower) to enable you to make that sacrifice. It really is going to depend on your acceptance and attitude toward what I have now deemed is necessary to say. I will have done you a gross injustice if I water down this message and tell you what you want to hear or what you are willing accept for your life. This is the basic message of truth, that *you are what you eat.* If you support your life living off dead, decaying manufactured, synthetic foods, then you may enjoy living as socially acceptable; but be assured of the reality that aging and parasitic diseases will eventually turn your life into a miserable existence, dependent on drugs, painkillers, medical care, and a prime candidate for an early grave. That's blunt truth, and older abused, depraved bodies cannot survive on synthetic foods for very long. The body's functions must have access to life-giving enzymes, minerals, and natural proteins to exist. Remember that all those wild days of drink and being merry have taken their toll on all our bodies' natural functions. Consuming toxins and preservatives over the years have overstressed those organs vital to maintaining good health and have created general confusion to our complex bodily functions that keep our lives operating in this overpopulated, polluted world. Most elderly people with chronic illnesses, sooner or later, give up on the life struggle and just want to go home peacefully to be with the Creator.

The oldies start to feel depressed and useless, believing they have nothing more to contribute to life. They may determine they are a burden to their loved ones and that nobody really cares one way or another whether they live or die. Their grown children are, in many cases, struggling to make ends meet, living and coping with the ever-growing difficulties of surviving in a debt-oriented society. They just don't have much time to devote to nurturing their elderly parents. Both parents are working to keep food on the table and taxes paid. Some kids see their parents on Christmas and birthdays. So many seniors get depressed with constant pain, both mental and physical, and start asking themselves why they should go on struggling to exist in this world when it appears that nobody really cares. This is a desperate, despondent mind-set and reveals an attitude of self-pity and low self-esteem. This condition is magnified by inactivity, poor health, low energy levels, and negative thoughts about growing older. Growing old is a natural function of life and has some great and wonderful benefits. The focus must not on the past but on the present. Looking back on my past life brings fond memories; however, that has nothing to do with my life in the present. I can't relive my past; but when I examine it objectively, I realize I lived with complete chaos and aimless directions, wondering the world over, driven and surviving by sheer instinct. I can now honestly say that for the first time in my life, I enjoy having clear, complete direction and control over my life. I have truly suffered and struggled miserably all my life with attention deficit/hypertension disorder (ADHD).

Any self-inflicted condition of boredom, depression, and despondency will change drastically as soon as your body and mind is functioning properly again; and real purpose is reinstated into your mind, life, and spirit. As our bodies become energized, and active life takes on renewed purpose and meaning. Excitement and positive attitudes are again reinstated back into our lives. It all starts with directing your thoughts and actions on obtaining spiritual awakening and optimum health at all cost. Believe me, living a healthy life without pain and anxiety will give your existing years on this planet a whole new meaning. Your options are very simple. You can let a disease-ridden, polluted environment terminate your desire to live, or you can take an optimistic leap of faith and take control of your life and health by living one day at a time. It is totally within your grasp to control your own health and spiritual destiny. It's a choice only you can make. I can, however, try to encourage you to find something close and dear to your life that will cause you to put forth the efforts needed to live a healthy, productive life again. Age has very little to do with your physical condition, but environment and mental attitude has everything to do with health. Don't blame the natural process of growing old for your condition of poor health. Look around, and you will see hundreds of seniors taking care of themselves and enjoying healthy and beneficial lives. What gives you the right to make old age your excuse for dropping out of our society?

I like to offer one more additional aid in helping you with this vital decision. What we senior citizens are suffering from is what I called old-age syndrome.

We are fading out of the mainstream of life, and we are being left out of the mainstream of world events. We oldies are no longer revered and respected by the new generations. We are being put in homes and sanctuaries for culling out of the society. Even with years of experience of living on this planet, we are no longer respected. In my opinion, never before in the history of this world has mankind needed the wisdom, experience, counseling, and influence from its older generations. With the world growing in chaos, insanity of leadership, weapons of mass destruction everywhere, and the uncertainty of the powerful, greedy world managers groping for world control, the future of mankind is very dubious. This new generation has not experienced or enjoyed true peace or real freedom. They have never lived in an environment where you could leave your home unlocked as crime was a novelty, not the expected. People respected the rights of persons to express themselves as they so desired. Television was unbiased news, and entertainment not polluted with violence and sex directed at undermining the Christian principles that form this nation. We, the freedom-loving Americans, have been supporting no-win wars somewhere on this planet for over twenty years. We have established military bases in over a hundred and twenty countries. What is that all about? Where is our young citizens whom we leave to manage this world, going to find and experience the knowledge, wisdom, and stability needed to deter and solve the incoming world disasters? Experienced men of peace are needed to confront and deal with the earth-shaking events and changes that the world is presently undergoing.

Freedom is being challenge to the core, and our world is being confronted with the greatest social challenges in its entire history. The very existence of mankind living on this planet is being constantly threatened with weapons of mass destruction. We have sat back and enjoyed our prosperity and peace, not realizing that opposing forces were about to create fear and apathy for the masses while slowly taking control of our planet's resources. The reason for controlling resources is simple. He who prints the money controls who gets the money. The drama that is presently being played out in the controlled media directed at our children is totally foreign to their experience and beyond their understanding. How are they going to deal with the fears and uncertainty of living in a world of perpetual wars, terrorism, and economic instability? It is my deepest conviction that our wisdom, stability, comfort, and experience will offer them the hope, incentive, and direction needed to make those life-sustaining choices that will be essential to dealing with this present world of insanity. Where else can they find the love and compassion needed to deal with the changes taking place in the family units of our world today? Have you not witnessed the total change in the makeup of our new generations of kids entrusted with the responsibility to take control of this world we leave them? As world events start to get totally unpredictable with unseen forces, creating total instability and uncertainty in the family unit, children will need our support and wisdom to give them vision and direction to make those vital decisions that will preserve life on this planet. That should help you to make the choice to live with a good quality of life.

Our present populations are being starved and deprived of the influence and exposure to godly qualities and influences that were the foundation of our present societies. Who is there left in this present world to carry on that godly social order that molded our country, once loved and respected by all the world populations and not feared? Where are those keepers of peace, liberty, and God? I feel deeply that aided with our support, stability, and experience, our next generation just might be able to deal with that godless uncertainty that is the signature of these present times. We have a monstrous task ahead of us, keeping sanity and spiritual meaning the main focus of life experience for our children and those yet unborn. We owe this to our parents who build this great nation on the principles that we the people are in trusted into the hands of God.

Obtaining and sustaining optimum health should not have to be a price tag. However, you will certainly pay a price in tenacity and vigilance that it will take to keep your life on the fast track. You are combating a constant barrage of elements and pollution being developed with overpopulation and industrial overload that is stressing out the planet we live in. Therefore, you will have to work a little overtime to keep the impact of environmental meltdown from stressing out your immune system. It should be a vital part of your inalienable right and a privilege of every person to have access to known and documented treatments for any potential disease and all vital public information needed to improve, sustain, and develop optimum health. Your government's job should be to protect its people from scams that feed off the ill health of our older populations.

That includes protection from drug cartels whose products are not designed to cure disease but to treat symptoms, for it's well-known that a person cured is a customer lost. Drugs, for the most part, are created for use-dependency, not to eliminate the causes and the effects of the disease. Symptoms may be put in remission with drugs, but making one "feel better" is not a cure. This is way short of what I would call restoring one's health; this is in effect being sold into bondage and dependency to the legal drug industry.

In most cases that I have witnessed, people have the capability of treating themselves inexpensively and effectively as long as they are offered the right information from their doctors, naturopaths, biochemists, and others humanitarians who value human life more than the almighty dollar. We may be living longer due to easier lifestyles, but is our quality of life better? Look at the statistics and visual evidence that will bear witness to more new diseases, obesity, and sickness in our society than ever before in our history. There is an epidemic out there witnessed by the billions, and billions of dollars are spent on medical and drug expenses. This little book will address the need for free souls to take responsibility for their own physical condition and their own health. It is written to encourage readers to take responsibility for their health and welfare to rid themselves of any condition that could be destroying their right to full and productive life. By this statement, I mean our lives should be in control of all forms of parasites that find our bodies delightful to live in. It is part of your inalienable rights to be able to maintain your own health on God's planet. That information is available in this book, so be prepared to take control.

The truths on natural, newly developed, proven health cures that are constantly being developed and marketed to the public on the Internet would be next to impossible to find in the medical media. It takes megabucks to buy TV time, advertising in the news media, or exposure in the mainstream media that's needed to expose the natural cures that are available to mankind today. These elite groups of enlightened natural health advocates are mostly underfunded, discredited, and have no means to reach the mass human market. Often, they are discredited and harassed by the government's protection agencies (FDA, AMA, etc.) that are on the large drug companies' payrolls. The synthetic drug industry has control of the mass media with their high cost of advertisement. The general public is constantly under bombardment with cleverly devised advertisement that is directed at programming our brains with the thinking your cure is only with your doctor. Then they are required by law to give you all the side effects of their drugs, which don't seem very important unless you're pregnant, have liver problems, headaches, high blood pressure, and the list goes on and on. The drug companies are making billions on their drugs, going direct to consumers with their promotion: "Go to your doctor and see if *painless* is right for you." Do you have any idea how expensive it is to buy prime time between seven and nine at night? All that promotion must be paying off big-time. Notice there's not a word about the cause or the cure for the disease. "See your doctor and ask if the purple pill is good for you." Doctors are also victims of the controlled medical system. Doctors start out wanting to help folks until they get into the game; then their minds get programmed by the system.

Their degree is contingent on them, following protocols and laws that allow them to become licensed to practice on the public. Many have seen through the fouled system and tried to change their ways by including natural remedies but are quickly reprimanded and forced back into the fold. It really comes down to choices. Unfortunately, most doctors remain in the system because it is very prestigious, very lucrative, and a billion-dollar system that has the resources to protect its control over all our health industry.

I realize that these statements are exposing some of the most powerful and established rituals in our so-called medical society, but we are now talking about your life and how to deal with its existence on this polluted planet. I am sorry but I have studied and documented many people that have taken back the responsibility of their own health. They have proven time after time that we have the ability to cure ourselves by using the path of natural treatments that God sanctions and endorses. *"If you can catch something, you can get rid of it" mentality.* That's where we are going in this book. It is my firm conclusion, and I pray yours, that there exists in nature a natural cure for every form of disease on the planet. It's time for you to start believing in God's nature's cures and his laws that govern all life on this planet. You were not created to endure pain and suffering. Seek with me that vital, enlightened awareness that God is truly working within you to fulfill the purpose of your creation. You are never alone in this pursuit of optimum health. As a final thought and reminder, no remedy fits all bodies, and each created person has its own formula for getting well. That's why we put God into the equation.

Boy, was that a long winded preface to this book. The rest of the book should go a lot faster and less personal. I just had a few things to get off my chest as I'm tired of no one addressing the issues that our nation is facing now. Hopefully, I will assist you in getting a better perspective of where we are going with the rest of the text of this book. We are facing exciting times, and I want to be there to witness all of it and maybe contribute some wisdom and experience to the godly solutions that will by necessary to take place. *It's call the fittest will survive.*

Congress shall make no law respecting an establishment of religion, or prohibiting the free exercise thereof; or abridging the freedom of speech, or of the press; or the right of the people peaceably to assemble, and to petition the government for a redress of grievances.

I gave an oath to protect that freedom, and this book, is an expression and exercise of that right. Statements I make are from my grievances against the ignorant practices that are prevalent in our health industry from men motivated by their pursuit of money and power.

Chapter 1

You Are What You Eat

I HAVE TO start this book by attacking a probably well-established gut set on the subject of food consumption. Odds are I will hit a very well-rooted brick wall of denial that has been fired into your mind-set from the beginning of your journey on planet earth. For you to agree and accept my plea for you to make the drastic changes in your eating habits will not get me votes. I am going to insist you concur and apply an earth-shaking and mind-boggling change in your lifestyle. This chapter could very well be the end of my creditability and relationship with you as my curious readers. I would only ask that you hear me out as I open my case and soul to the issues set before you. Give me a little slack to ramble on so I can share some of the convictions I have acquired for my life and am now religiously applying to what's left of my sojourn on this planet. Having traveled this planet for seventy-eight years, I might just be able to help you avoid some of the damage that I have done to my health. We humans, for the security and enjoyment of belonging to the world herd, have become creatures of customs, apathy, traditions, and media hogwash. We feed off the so-called manufactured foods that our taste buds have been programmed and trained to enjoy. We are creatures of habits, good and bad. The so-called health experts have determined what foods are good for us and what form of nourishment we need for our bodies. The mass media is being used by the massive food industry into programming our minds into believing we are living to eat, and that eating is a social function that has become a form of pastime entertainment.

That's only a part of their program. Behind that fast-food industry is the synthetic food manufactures who financed and propagated the greatest exploration of dead toxic food this world has ever witnessed. They take a beautiful God; create natural food product; dry it; grind it; color it; preservative it; put it in a box, can, or bottle; and sell it worldwide as food. It's distributed and placed on the store shelves for months until the some naive consumers buy it for food. The corporate system of food production sells and distributes billions of pounds of the synthetic substance worldwide that feeds the majority of the world's advanced societies. Every society that has open trade agreements with the United States have our manufactured foods impacting into their marketplaces all over their nations. I was working in Costa Rica for years and witnessed their government protecting our corporate American interests in that they were building monster shopping malls and bringing in their corporate, processed canned foods that were geared to a shelf life of mega years. I have been privilege to be able to travel all over the world, and I could always buy a canned food or find a box of cornflakes. These small sovereign nations have lost total control of their economic futures as corporate America has totally undermined their local food consumption customs. They are now serving their populations with our addictive foods and sweets. Their cultures have been undermined with well-planned programs to turn their populations into addicted consumers of the fast-food industrialists. Their children are being saturated with advertisements, changing their eating habits to that of their idols in the American society.

The free import and export programs are just a legal license for corporate America to rape and pilferage their nation's economies. All the new industrial nations are indebted to the world bankers and must open their markets to the American industrial conglomerate. Their governments are helpless to protect their populations as we use their cheap labor to work in our factories to produce the fast-food industry. I was living in Costa Rica and had a big American factory opened up right down from my factory where I was making sidings, four-inch-by-eight-foot sheets for my steel homes I was building. They were building their homes in concrete block, and the country sits right on a fault line and shakes constantly, putting a strain on their cement homes especially the peonies building on public lands bordering rivers. With no foundations, their homes would end up in the bottom of the canyon as they were rigid and heavy. My steel homes were flexible and are today 90 percent of the homes being built in Costa Rica.

The outcome of this travesty is human bodies all over the world are experiencing various new health disorders never before seen or encountered. I call this tragedy "the dead food conspiracy." It is worldwide epidemic that is growing leaps and bounds. When we send aid to a starving nation, it is not in the form of food that they have been accustomed to consuming, it is in a can. I have seen the cooks dress it up with all their natural herbs. I saw this in Spain, France, and Germany as I lived there for years.

The third world nations have been victims of the corporate world food-processing agenda for years as I have witnessed it firsthand. We are well in the process of changing the eating habits of the entire world populations.

No human body is immune or safe from the natural reactions from eating deadly synthetic, toxic foods. The sugar-infested, habit-forming fast-food industry have opened their hamburger, coffee, ice cream, supermarkets, and joints all over the world – thanks to the intimidation of our corporate-controlled government. You see, folks, we have our peace-keeping troops embedded in a hundred and twenty countries out of a hundred and sixty odd that exist. Who is picking up that little tab? If you're not ticked off at your so-called representative government, you should be.

There is now a growing group of well-informed human souls living in the security of their homes who have opted out of the corporate food supply chain and are growing or purchasing natural-grown, organic foods. Foods that God has created just for mankind to protect and sustain a natural, normal existence on his planet. We all must take control of what we eat as nourishment and not offer our bodies up as victims to the fast-food cartels. In short, it is your responsibility to maintain the life that has been given you and to see that it receives the natural foods that God created it to survive on. If your body dies prematurely, then you have no one to blame but yourself. The life entrusted to your actions is one of your God-given responsibilities. Animals instinctively know how and what to eat to sustain their lives. The giant corporate food manufacturers have created the ultimate system of processed foods. They have designed, established, and documented how they now have fast foods that will stand on store shelves almost indefinitely. They have cloned the original flavors of their products into a near-perfect, synthetic copy of the natural flavors.

If they can't copy the original flavor, they certainly can create a new flavor that is proven and tested to give your taste buds a more pleasant experience. I don't think for one minute that so-called food being sent by the tons to those rogue nations in trouble is anything like the culinary enjoyment they are accustomed to eating? What a wonderful opportunity to dump a lot of outdated processed foods as undesirables. I wonder why our government hasn't considered trading food for oil. Boy, you can bet the drug moguls will be sending in there acid reflex pills and a lot of Tums for the tummy. One bullet they dodged is government can't send in a lot of ice cream as they don't have reliable sources of refrigeration. Boy, if you can't beat them, poison them with the food. Could I have fun with this, but I won't. I hope you will agree with me that mankind is not capable of creating a synthetic form of food that can compete in nutritional values that God has designed into his natural foods grown to sustain our lives on earth.

As you can now detect, my first approach to good health is eating as much, if not all, of your food in its natural state – raw. This means you must first start rejecting those foods that do you the most harm and need sugar to make it palatable. If you are not convinced, I know what I am talking about, just hang in there and remain open-minded. I have been labeled a health freak by my fellow actors as I consume over 80 percent of my food in its natural state. Not many of my golfing buddies like hearing my radical convictions on health practices, but a lot of those youngsters can't beat this seventy-eight-year-old handicap man. The changing of my eating habits has made a drastic change in my life.

I made up my mind after extensive research and viewing documented evidence that eating living food in its natural state was imperative if I was going to receive the necessary nourishments needed to keep my body alive and kicking at my age. Most all processed foods having been infested with chemicals and toxins are a total drain on our immune systems. The synthetic food industry not only has created habit-forming foods for the public but are the primary contributors to obesity and disease that's running rampant throughout our society. What has happened to our public awareness, revealing that the food we consume is for the purpose of sustaining life, receiving nourishment and the energy needed to enjoy our lives? This is a normal function of our bodies to eat to live by consuming natural foods in their natural state. This order in life seems to have been nullified or rendered meaningless by our media-controlled society who dances to the tune of their clients. Did you know that it takes huge amounts of energy and over four hours to digest the processed foods we eat? Remember it has been cooked, saturated with preservatives, and packed in a vacuum. Your body's digestive process has to go through a massive breakdown ritual just to find something beneficial for your life force. If your body could talk to you, it would shout out and clear your brain-dead idiot when it comes to selecting food to sustain your life. That is substantiated by the nostalgic, tired feelings our body's witness after consuming a large synthetic meal. It is time you realize that your body is using up more energy trying to digest that garbage than the benefits it receives from that tedious digestive process. Your body is now on that slippery slop to the grave.

When the body starts to accumulate and store all those foreign additives, preservatives, dyes, toxins, and fillers – thinking it's nourishment to be used at a later date – the body doesn't consider that your brain doesn't know the difference between its natural foods and corporate garbage. The storing of that garbage in our bodies is easily detected and reflected in the gaining of weight, less energy, more susceptible to disease ailments, stress, and depressed mental attitude. This, along with low self-esteem, is prominent in major percent of our populations. Over 75 percent of our population is obese, with that figure growing faster among our children. The real evidence in this growing deficiency in our society is the growing need for a quick energy fix from the thousands of sugar-based foods available everywhere you look. The next time you grab a tasty synthetic treatment, just look on the label and see if it contains a form of sugar. Sugar-based foods are not the foods that God has designed to support your daily energy requirements. The food that one eats must contain sustaining types of natural nourishment to produce energy that can last for hours. The body needs constant flow of energy distributed by the blood to reach and supply every cell in the body. Not a sugar fix that offer highs and lows with a toxic hangover. Eat natural foods that offer live enzymes, minerals, and vitamins that have time to release qualities. They are easier dissimulated as they are naturally grown and designed by our Creator for human consumption. They can be digested and put into use within an hour after consumption and will sustain our life force for many hours. Fruits take an even shorter periods of time for us to digest.

The farmers who produce all-natural foods needed to sustain our lives don't have large cooperative structures behind them to market and advertise their goods. Why should they have to compete for your dollar at the marketplace against the mega large fast-food industry? Did you notice that 90 percent the foods in the grocery stores are produced by corporate food conglomerates and that the natural organic foods are only located in one small corner of the store. The farmers of America have been our only source of life-giving natural foods for two hundred years. Should we abandon them to support the new corporate food industries? They are still the organic food growers at the local grocery stores. I don't think so. Take a positive action and look to support the organic food industry for the benefit of your health. By buying natural-grown veggies, nuts, and fruits, the natural enzymes will produce changes in your health, eating habits, and your taste buds. Natural cereals, soy milk, fruits, raw honey, and orange juices for breakfast will start your day with nature's best offerings to preserve your life. The consumption of live, natural foods instead of dead, processed food will make a big difference in your overall health. You might start the pursuit of optimum health by bringing your weight under control. Now let's have a look at another aspect of the eating foods that are designed for you bodies. You realize, of course, the food you eat produces nutrients that must be used, eliminated, or stored by the body as they have to go somewhere. Manufactured complex foods require a more complex and long digestive process. A manufactured product has a lot of chemicals that are not readily useable for the body.

Processing this complex material overloads the organs, and mainly the liver, as it is the principal organ we rely on to cleanse the body of toxins and aid in the digestive process. Do you know that we can carry around five to forty pounds of fecal matter in our intestinal tracts as undigested, putrefied matter? Have you noticed all the little potbellies running around with thin body parts? The intestinal track is an awful place to store unwanted food particles, and you need to have a gut cleanse on a regular schedule. The decayed fecal matter makes and gives off toxins, gases, and other odors that are very noticeable when you sweat and poop. Any toxic, indigestible junk food is a great breeding place for all parasites that developed other forms of disease. It has been said that most diseases start in our intestinal tract and are carried to other parts of the body by the bloodstream. In fact, it's documented that we all can have the cancer cells propagating years before it becomes prevalent to our systems. They essentially start their degenerating process in our intestinal tracts and then migrate to any weak organ or another component in our body (*http://www.askdrkelly.com/*).

Without the proper elimination of all unused *foreign fecal matters* that are preservatives, chemicals, minerals, and toxins, you are creating gigantic problems for your immune system. The body normally assumes that you instinctively know what natural foods it needs to function properly, but looking at today's menus, nothing is further from the truth. What your body needs and what you are feeding it may have nothing in common. All the additives corporate food industry using in the making of synthetic foods directed at entrapping your taste buds is working.

Is it any wonder that the overall health condition of our populations are in subnormal condition as witnessed by the massive trillion-dollar medical and drug industry that nobody addresses? Do you realize that most human bodies subjected to this abuse are now operating under tremendous stress, struggling constantly to obtain the nourishment the body needs to exist on our polluted planet? Over 50 percent of our populations have some form of chronic illnesses. Stop and think about that for a minute, what natural food did you feed your body today that would support its daily need to maintain optimum running condition for today? May I demonstrate a small part of what I am talking about? I might refer to couple of popular choices that many uninformed victims of the fast-food industry make on a daily basis. Such as a Coca-Cola for quenching thirst, candy bars for quick nourishment, pork sausage for protein, and processed white breads for seeds and grains. We stuff ourselves on wonderful-tasting denatured stuff that has to been seasoned to make it palatable, cooked till it has nothing of value left in it, and placed on the shelf until it is well seasoned. We are literally starving our bodies into an early death. I am a radical for sure, but my body at seventy-eight doesn't lack of nourishment to keep it afloat and in good optimum health. The fast-food industry is constantly developing more sophisticated synthetic foods for man to consume. Did you know that some foods contain minute particles of minerals and preservatives that the FDA will classify as natural ingredients? That's great. Maybe if you only take it once or twice a week, you will live a few weeks longer.

It's like playing Russian roulette with your life force. What if it only makes you a little sick? Now you can become addicted and don't have to worry as you're going to die in any case. Of course some of the processed foods, not digestible, will build up and become stored in your system for later use. Good luck as your body doesn't realize you have no use for synthetic foods that are overcooked and nutrient-dead. This doesn't include the harm you are causing your digestive system. The solution is simple. Stop looking on the shelves of the marketplace for nourishment to keep your body in the game of living on this planet as you won't find it there. You must trot over to that small fresh food produce department and purchase those living organic foods that produce the nourishment, vitality, and longevity in your life God has created just to sustain you life force.

What really amazes me is that people would never consider putting kerosene fuel into their automobiles that require unleaded gas, but they have very little or no concern for the damage they are doing to their bodies by consuming synthetic, dead foods from fast-food markets. Most people take better care of their cars than they do their bodies. Do I not sound like some far-out radical who is pounding the pavement on an issue that's destroying the world's populations? Well, I'm totally convinced that before you go making a commitment to seek a hundred years of disease-free life, you had better check the odds and look at the evidences. It can be done, but it takes a certain amount of dedication to eating natural foods in their natural state – raw. Foods designed to keep our lives in tune with our body's life force. Seek a hundred years of healthy life by lining up with God's program.

Only natural program that brings that goal into the realm of reality is the living nutrients that your blood carries to all your vital organs. We have to start with considering the application of a proven commonsense approach to all our eating habits. We can't stop the deterioration of aging to our bodies until we accomplish the replenishing of all the vital elements and nutrients that keeps those body functions operating at optimum performance. Adjustments are needed now, and commitments made to make the radical changes in our food consumption especially if you're eating from the corporate food trough. You know, one vital functions of your immune system is being unconsciously engaged in keeping your life on top of earth and your heart strong in the game of serving your body needs with life-giving nutrients. When those organs are no longer receiving the needed nourishments from your blood supply, they start to cease function properly, and the body suffers. Because your stomach is full doesn't mean you are getting the nourishment needed to keep you alive and kicking. Common sense has to tell you that your poor choices in food consumption are the determining factors in sustaining your life on this planet. You can choose the foods that support your life functions, or you can eat the foods that your taste buds have been programmed to enjoy that offer you an early exit from earth. The choice is yours. Eat what the nutritionist say is vital nourishment for your body's survival or eat the synthetic fast-food garbage that the fast-food moguls who don't give a damn about your health make available at your local grocery store. Addictive foods have been created with sweets to program the taste buds of uninformed public who feed at the corporate trough.

They take advantaged of their clients with appealing ads and devious assumptions that they are getting the best food money can buy. The public as a whole are uninformed as to what foods are compatible and needed for his digestive system to sustain the life force in his body. Do you have any idea how much of our populations are running about stressed out with undernourished bodies? You will join that joyful crowd that's supporting the drug industry existing of aspirins, Tums, peptic, and other drugs designed to keep the body comforted while being stressed out on its feet. Then down the line, it all catches up with us, and we go into total overload and vitality rundown. Disease attacks every weakness from the heart to having run-down organs in our body. Now we shift into save-the-life mode and are forced to take on any means of treatment that the medical gurus determine will sustain our lives. I was just informed today that one of my close golfing buddies has inoperable pancreatic cancer. There is no medical solution for this disease in the massive, controlled drug industry. Try to tell that to Dr. Kelley at *http://www.askdrkelly.com/*, "One Answer to Cancer." Read his account of how he cures himself of pancreatic cancer and hundreds of others.

I just did a little test on myself as to the validity of my words. I just had breakfast at the golf club. You know what I ate? Biscuits with pork gravy and eggs with hash browns. My stomach is now turning cartwheels, and you should have seen the other choices on the menu. My golfing partners think I'm weird eating fruit for snacks on the course instead of candy bars and soda pop. Did I say it would be easy for you to make lifestyle food adjustments?

Determine for yourself right now if you want to live in harmony with the natural functions of your body? Are you going to strive to feed your body the foods that it was designed by the Creator to sustain your life on this planet? Just how important is your health, and do you want to live to be a hundred? If you continue to live in the mainstream of the food guzzlers of this society, you have sealed your own doom. Are you laughing at this statement? Then you are not ready to make overall commitment to eating all proper foods that God intended you to consume. Sure, you can fall back and taste foods you become addicted to, but don't rely on them to sustain your life. In time you will lose the desire to eat those dead foods, and your habits will change and take on a totally different direction.

There are many new species of virus and bacteria being introduced every day into the public herd. Some are in our foods with new taste bud delights being made available by the food industry. Some are deadly and mysterious as the medical system has very little control over the food industry. Hundreds more are becoming immune to the drugs and antibiotics that the drug corporations are creating. You're either going to eat the live foods that your body needs, or you're going to be a victim or a statistic of a short resident on our planet. Your overworked, undernourished immune systems will deteriorate into the pits if not looked after. Your chances of enjoying optimum health will be slim and none if you're not on top of looking after your body. Sounds like I'm beating a dead horse, but if I don't take a positive attitude toward looking after your health, then nothing else I have to say will make any sense.

You really need to hear and listen to that small voice of common sense in your subconscious mind that whispers loud and clear every time you take a drink or eat a mouthful of factory-produced shelf food. "You are what you eat." If I can make you conscientious about how, when, and what you partake for your food consumption, then my labors are not in vain. My last offering on this matter, if you're not feeding your body with what it can digest and use for nourishment, then your are feeding hundreds of different species of parasites that are enjoying your meal.

The body is documented to carry over four hundred known species of parasites. We will address this subject in detail later.

Let's talk now about protein and its vital value to our lives. High protein consumers smell to high heaven as the overload toxins are being released through the skin when the temperature rises above body temperature. We know many scientific studies have been conducted by certain biased interests. The meat suppliers have made their studies, and the soybean growers have done their share, and the controversy goes on and on. Who do you believe? You believe your body and mind (eat@veat.com). Who are our closest relatives in the animal kingdom? Apes and monkeys! Their diet is mainly fruit nuts. What foods do most humans on earth eat that is universally enjoyed? Fruit and nuts. The world's consumption of fruit exceeds any other food source by the majority of populations on this planet. That's a commonsense application of what you should eat as the main staple to sustain your life force.

Meat eaters have a very unique characteristic that sets them apart from all the rest of the animal kingdom.

First, they have short, smooth digestive tracts like a pipe; and their digestive juices are acidic. They have no problem digesting high cholesterol and have no need of fiber to move fecal matter through their short digestive tracts. The adult human digestive tract averages over twenty-seven feet and is bumpy and filled with pockets. He needs fiber, and his juices are alkaline that helps him predigest plant foods. The reason for this is his food of choice should be fruits as fruits decay very rapidly and is readily assimilated into the body. The carnivores have short digestive tracks and release ten times more hydrochloric acid to digest fiber, blood, and bones. They also don't sweat except though their tongues, so they hunt at night and sleep during the heat of the day. And we do not need to emphasize the difference between the teeth of a lion and that of a human. It suffices to say flesh eaters don't have molars to grind food. They have long pointed fangs to rip and tear their prey.

In conclusion, we are not equipped to be carnivores, but in fact, we are herbivores. We have to cook the meat we eat so that we can devour it with little effort and make it more digestible to our system. We use spices and sauces to make meat palatable and enjoyable to eat. Meat is not made for human consumption as we are herbivores and have no teeth to tear meat of the carcass of a beef cow.

When one considers that flesh foods of all kinds are extremely toxic, it becomes apparent that they should be labeled as an extremely undesirable form of nourishment for our bodies. In the eating of flesh, one must take into account all of our eliminative organs and their functions. They are made by our Creator to treat the ingestion of vegetables and fruits.

When we add animal flesh containing the excessive proteins and fats (drugs and other unusable chemicals are also prevalent), extra labor is required by our digestive systems in dealing with the toxic matter. Remember that all foods must be broken down into a liquid form to be digested and distributed by your blood to all parts of your body. Nutrients siphoned from the flesh (including fish) take hours longer to reach a state of liquidity before they are beneficial to the body functions. I just ate an organic hamburger, and my stomach went into convulsions. Just thought I could get by with eating a little organic ground-up meat, I was wrong; so I'm back on fruits, vegetables, and Pepto-Bismol just to stop the belching. (Read Stanley Burroughs.) Just another professional opinion that makes a case for the consumption of natural-grown foods stronger.

Charles Darwin, who offered the theory of evolution, has declared that humans are fruit and vegetable eaters throughout the history of our anatomy. Maybe now is the time for you to reevaluate your eating habits. Do you think it is possible for you to rethink and adjust your selecting foods that you feed your body? Is it possible you could make an effort to change poor habits that have been instilled into you from birth? Could you make this choice even on a conditional basis? Could you allow a common logical sense evaluation be the salvation of your life to take control over your eating habits? I would now strongly suggest reading the book *Fit for Life* by Harvey and Marilyn Diamond. I am not trying to be an inspirational writer that is playing mind games with your brain as I leave that up to our government stooges. I just desire you to consider my findings.

I hope I am able to convince you to make this dedicated, lifesaving adjustment to your life. "The herb of the field shall be thy meat" "Let thy food be thy medicine, and thy medicine be thy food" (Gen. 1:29). Hypocrites. There is so much wisdom in those words. A lot of times we know what to do, but are unable to do it as our minds and willpowers become weak and programmed with time. Old habits have taken control of our lives supported with the constant barrage of media blitz. We are being controlled by our macho-herd instincts and egos that proclaim a false sense of pride in being a big steak eater or booze drinker. I was in that trap for years. That socially acceptable and manly carnivorous pleasures of overeating high protein diets will certainly shorten your residence on this planet. If you could just see the host of parasites and chemicals that have become permanent residents in your body from the red meat you consume, I would win my case hands down. Why can't we seem to muster up the intestinal fortitude to separate ourselves from the herd of meat eaters? What does it take to convince you that you will not return to Eden with the blood of diseased animals running through your veins.

As long as we trod along with the human herd, we will succumb the dictates of its wranglers, the medical cartel. The prime examples are the alcoholics and drug addicts whose lives are totally lost in their addictions and their inability to help themselves. Their attempts to attend classes for rehabilitation have offered little or no success. He has found comfort in belonging to his own little herd of addicts. Millions of dollars are being spent trying to cure addicts with gimmicks when all that needed is a sincere commitment to God.

Seeking and receiving God's love will install a new self-image, a new person in Christ that transforms our souls, and we are a creation of God's grace and love. He loves us and will not abandon his creation to aimlessly wander over his planet. You may be desperate and addicted to self-destruction, but God cannot and will not turn his back on your cries of remorse and repentance. He is unable to intervene with your exercise of self-will, and accepting his love has to be an exercise of your free will. He waits your partition for his help. You have to overcome your own ego and humbly ask for God to intervene in your life. All we need to offer is the willingness to respond and become the object of God's affections. It is a belief system where we take God at his Word. God has expressed in his Holy Word that he is willing and able to cure any mental or physical disorders that prevent us from living in harmony with him and all his creation. The key to securing health starts in the heart and soul with a deep, sincere desire to serve and possess God's love. If God doesn't care and you are unable to experience his embracing love, then your life has no meaning as well as all creation about you. You see, nothing makes sense if the world did not have a creator and you are not part of that creation. Now you need to take a hard look at his creation and determine what kind of God preformed this task. I choose to look at the beauty in creation, and I witness a loving, caring God that placed us in an environment to prosper and enjoy a fulfilling life. My God, who reveals himself in all that he has created, is my role model in my hope and trust for the salvation of my soul. The relief from a vision of eternal separation from my Creator.

Obesity in man is the by-product of a diet out of control, a mind that is complacent, and a willpower that is dormant. It is also death trap and contributes to having a body supporting millions of unwanted parasites and toxins. You need to take this first step in your quest for optimum health very seriously. There is no set program I can give you that fits every life; therefore, every person must research and apply this important, life-altering decision for himself and on his or her own terms. The point I make is that you must make this choice for yourself at all costs. I can assure you that this is the most serious decision that you face other than God being the center force in your life. How close are you to giving this one gigantic step, the commitment of all your best efforts to accomplish?

Do you want to know how bad refined sugar is for you and your system? Look up *Sugar Blues* on the Net, and with half a brain, you will give up refined sugar for life. Once you have beat the acquired addictive sweet-tooth syndrome, the rest of the program starts to get easier depending on how addicted you have become and your commitment to restoring your optimum health. By starting small sacrifices like no candy bars, less sugar in your coffee, and giving up known eating habits that have excess sugar contents, you will be off the starting line to reversing your bodies' destiny with a miserable, premature death. Some of our siblings or weaklings may need to find some alternate natural food sources to replace the sugar cravings. Fruits and nuts are the best way to go to break the sugar blues, but for the sake of your future and self-esteem, don't cave in to your bad habits as it will put a real dent in your self-esteem.

You must believe in yourself to take control of your health because eating is a natural habit. Boy, am I profound it scares me. You are capable of keeping your commitment to yourself and building your eating habits up to the point of consuming living, vital, nourishing food for most of your intake of daily food consumption. You are going to start living in harmony with nature. You're going to stop being a victim of the fast, synthetic food industry. Stop trying to live off dead animals or their by-products. Look after your bodies' needs and functions and prepare to receive the blessings beyond your wildest dreams.

I now can assure you of one thing about eating to live. When we become accustomed to eating all-natural foods, we get a decisive change within our taste buds. The foods that were once repulsive to us become delightful flavors with herbs and flavors you have never witnessed before. Your tastes and senses will experience new enjoyments in eating that you couldn't dream would ever happen. You will love natural fruits, nuts, and the multitude of veggies used in salads with flavorful herbs and natural olive oils. You will taste things in foods that you have never sensed before. There will be a day that your life will no longer crave dead foods, and you will be turned on with the consuming of foods that your body is compatible with. The eating of natural foods will be a cuisine in eating and knowing you are in tune with the universe. What a relief to know you are feeding your body what it was designed by God to sustain your optimum health. Your food should be your medicine, and it should and does contain all the natural nourishments needed to maintain your optimum health.

The picture I enjoy painting is that of the guru that lives ageless in the Himalayas or the Okinawa men who have the longest life expectancy in the world. They have thirty-four men living over the age of a hundred out of every one hundred thousand men. In America, we have ten to every one hundred thousand. Just wanted you to see the odds that I am up against in my quest for a long, healthy life. I have twenty more years to go as most of my fellow TV cowboys are long gone. I believe it is the food they consumed that has caused their early retirement from our planet. If they had lived of fruits, veggies, herbs, and some fish, many of them might still be in the saddle.

Eating natural foods has to have some creditability and should certainly meet the test of being a part of commonsense approach to restoring natural living. We will see some positive results in any effort to align our eating habits with the master plan of God. I'm sure he created all those various fruits and veggies worldwide with you in mind. Are we not his created participants of his unconditional love and created in his image? Everything he created has order and meaning on this planet, and nothing has happened by chance. His creative intelligence created all the various life-forms that placed man at the heart of his creation.

Your health is the one thing you can create; and it is yours to restore, sustain, and implement. Am I getting your attention? Can you now start to see that I'm not beating a dead horse and that we are able to get on the right track to self-healing and living a rich and fulfilling life span? Depression will be an emotion in the past, and you will wake up every morning with a renewed energy, looking forward to each day with a renewed spirit of peace and love.

You will be looking for new things to get evolved with as your mind become alert and new energy flows throughout your body. All the vital parts are now working to a new rocky mountain high. There is so much we miss in this life when we exist with a depressed, depraved, malnourished body. Healthy lives bring on a healthy lifestyle that reflects in every aspect of your daily living, but it comes with a price. Many in the herd will not pay as we become attached to the human herd and don't like being different or living out of the mainstream of acquired customs. Eating at the human junk food trough is being in the mainstream of human behavior today. I know I am beating a dead horse, but if I can get you to make a commitment to take me serious and make a food consumption change in your eating habits, I have accomplished the impossible in your life. I would like to feel that I contributed something more than killing a few bad guys to the enjoyment of your life.

Another great advantage of eating healthy herbs and veggies is that obesity will be a nightmare in the past. You cannot overeat as the carbohydrates and animal fats do not exist in plants. Your body will naturally shut down when it is satisfied, and there is nothing in what you have eaten to store. You will not desire to eat more food as with the habit of meat consumption. I have seen people eat steaks by the numbers. I mean gorge on themselves with red meat. Why did they take the time to strip the skin of? Dead foods designed to entrap your taste buds will also produce a negative effect on your metabolism as they cannot satisfy your needs for life-giving nourishments. After eating a raw meat, your body may still be hungry for the nourishments.

The stomach enzymes may be maxed, trying to break down that cow flesh. In the meantime, our bodies are deprived of nourishment needed to do the job on the cow. Your body will probably adjust to the overload of dead food you ate, but it might need some sleep so it can concentrate its efforts on the cow you ate. Folks, I can assure you your body is being overworked trying to digest that cow you ate. It is loaded with toxic elements; it's working overtime at digesting flesh while seeking nourishment for the body. The body's reaction to unwanted foods, toxins, and liquids is by storing them all over your body in the form of lumps and fatty tissue. The body has no idea how foolish you are about your food consumption. One of the greatest reasons for heart failures is fatty tissue built up around the heart from unwanted food sources. The medics tell you that you have a cholesterol problem, but that is just a media-medical hype. The real problem is the type and quality of food we consume. Bringing your eating habits under your control, a giant step that has been taken, and you will see a difference in your health pursuit in short order.

The downside is some of you readers are addicted to junk food and will not ever make the grade to help your bodies achieve optimum health. The habits of eating certain dead foods have entrapped your taste buds and mind-set that will reject all common sense and will not prove facts on healthy eating habits. It sorts of reminds me of our politics of divide and conquer. Everything today has dual meanings. We can't find any weapons of mass destruction; terrorism is everywhere, and we need to blow up some terrorist nation that has been living peacefully for centuries before we existed.

We are using our young troops as cannon fodder for the world oil cartel. Who dares to question the validity of our government's troops who always has our best interest in heart? If Bush says that there were weapons of mass destruction, then there were weapons of mass destruction somewhere. You can see the planned divisiveness of dividing the confused populations of lemmings into believing their media hypes and half-truths.

That same process has been used within the health industry to the point where you don't know in whom to believe. *I'm simply saying that eat all-healthy, wholesome, natural foods. Let it be your medicines. That is the only path to optimum health. Eat foods that are alive, and stay alive.*

Other good readings are the following: *The Pro-Vita Plan* by Dr. Jack Tips, also *Nourishing Traditions* by Sally Fallon, and *The Metabolic Typing Diet* by William Wolcott and Trish Fahey.

Chapter 2

Energize Body and Mind

NOW WE ARE going to address an area of our health systems in my thinking that will release us from the bondage of apathy, complacency, stubbornness, insecurity, and bad habits. We have been psyched, programmed, and duped by the cleverly orchestrated media hype into being the subjects and supporters of the lifeless products of the dead food industry. There is a giant worldwide industry in place that has entrapped most of the world's populations into becoming willing victims of garbage foods and sweet, polluted drinks industry that have developed into the historic desecration of the human race.

We are being subjected to a constant barrage of media publicity selling the synthetic dead foods created by the corporate giants that have customized and victimized the inhabitants of this world with eating their manufactured toxic foods. Boy, I bet you're tired of hearing that. They say repeating oneself over again shows the importance in the topic. You just can't imagine the amount of profit that's built into that little candy bar. The one that sits behind the cashier's desk, indefinitely waiting for some sweet-addicted victim to scoop it up and try to find some nourishment out of it to sustain his life. That's what we eat food for, isn't it?

It's certainly not the small farmers, almost extinct on this continent, that are to blame. It is corporate growers who now controls the mass production of our stressed-out food supply. These large corporate-growing machines have purchased large tracts of our farmlands and put the small farmers out of business. They have turned the farmlands into a massive food-producing industry, hiring illegal emigrants, using pesticides and growth fertilizers to enhance the productivity and, in turn, create more profit. The products of sugar, wheat, and other foods produced are then dried, burned, grounded, mixed, added with preservatives, colors, tastes, sugars, and chemicals and packed them into a can, bottle, bag, or package, and put into the marketplace. Some are processed and canned and placed on the shelves of our markets and then referred to as food. They are notorious for hiring cheap illegal aliens to work the land and cultivate their crops that have been grown with chemical fertilizers and pesticides. These industrial giants of the food industry are a massive force that has taken on the responsibility of supplying our food.

The general public totally depends on the quality, pureness, and affordability of the massive food industry to feed and maintain the general health and welfare of all the world populations of today. We freedom lovers, who are trusting and benevolent and believes in God, are convinced that our food source is being protected by our government. That we are being protected by our government and its many agencies from any harmful products that could endanger the lives of our citizens. Nothing is further from the truth. Did you know that they are now radiating the food we feed our children at schools? What's new? Read

"The Ducuypere Report" (healthalternatives.com). *This is only a small part of the picture.*

California's produce industry is an example of the corporate food industries' mass concentration of food production for fruit, nuts, and vegetables grown on prime land. The San Joaquin Valley seldom lies dormant as it is in constant production. It uses massive amounts of pesticides, foreign pickers, and fertilizers to grow and develop their continuous need for producing products. I would just like to mention to you that some of these pesticides and fertilizers used by the growers to produce massive amounts of food for U.S. markets. This information is offered in order for you to see how important it is to combat the side effects our bodies are suffering from the constant intake of these radiated foods. First, there are insecticides such as diazinon, oxamyl, etc. Second, we have the herbicides Paraquat, Oryzalin, etc. And third, we have nematicides, such as Telone, Varlex, etc., And last but not the least, what is used in our orchards is rodenticides.

All these additives and sprays are sanctioned by your government, and all are potentially deadly to mankind. Eating one or two of these pesticides may not kill you, but consuming them on a steady diet will certainly accumulate in your body and cause you a lot of damage down the line. Your body will eventually become overloaded with the toxins and deadly foreign matter stored, and you'll die. You do not have any idea how much of these chemical additives we are accumulating every time as we consume a hot dog at the fast-food dispensary. There are organic pesticides available to farmers; however, they are only used by a small group of organic growers as they are not cost-effective to the food globalists who have another agenda in mind.

If those added chemical products will kill bugs, rats, fungus, and whatever else is feeding of our food source, then it certainly can't be considered safe for us *Homo sapiens* who are further up the food chain. Tell me, is it more important to have the product looking good or to have it safe to eat? What in God's name is the accumulation of those additives going to do in our bodies? What is their effect on our bodies from a long-term consumption, not considering the unknown pollutions from handling the stuff with deterioration and storing? Are we not the most trusting souls alive to support and believe in a system that has one purpose in life: make money. Boy, I'm totally convinced humans are self-inflicted victims to apathy, ignorance, and naivety. Our food source should be the most protected and coveted industry in our society. People should not have to die before we find something wrong with any particular product.

All foods, and I mean all foods, should have to be organically grown with no exceptions. That's a little price to pay for consuming a safe product. There I go again trying to live in a perfect environment in a failed, greedy, decaying, and money-orientated system. It just wouldn't be cost-effective, would it? And worst, the medical and drug cartel would lose millions in revenue. We all know we should always trust our corporate-run government agencies that are diligently looking after the health and welfare of their vast populations of sheeplings. I wonder who is looking after big governments and making sure they are serving the interests of us little people and not their mentors, the corporate food giants. We the people pay their salaries, but corporate world pays for their perks for living high off the hog. I guess, the real answer to what they make is private and only the Internal Revenue Service (IRS) knows what they file as truth. Boy, I'm not going there as I found very little on the Net that gives a definitive answer to that question. We can be assured that our honorable servants are on only a few corporate payrolls. It's not a perfect system, is it? But it also is not getting any better with time. I feel it's time to take control of your life as it doesn't look like your government gives a hoot about your health and welfare. I can promise you that the handful of elites who sit on the seats of the one-world government would like to see the populations of this world culled to more than half of what it is today.

How did the medical industry become such a multitrillion-dollar business in such a short period of time? I mean, in my lifetime, they have gone from being a family doctor making house calls to a multitrillion-dollar rip-off of the American people.

It is truly a giant corporate structure that has taken over of the medical needs of the entire populations of the world from an office building. There are new diseases emerging, spreading everywhere with discoveries of new viruses and bugs being a constantly exposed to our societies. It's almost like someone is working full-time to come up with new diseases so that the drug industries can come up with a new treatments that siphon billions out of the naive victims of the pill cartel. It sure wasn't that way when I was a little fellow living and working on my grandfather's farm in Austin, Texas. That was the age when the doctors were friends of the natural cures, made house calls, and delivered babies at home. The biggest problems we faced as kids were treated – a cold, small pox, or poison ivy. Something has transpired that is no longer in tune with nature or God as money has replaced care and concern for the less fortunate who are victims of a contaminated planet. Did you know that there are at least twenty known different chemical sprays that are being used to control pests on farm products and in the orchards of our country? Over 1.5 billion pounds of pesticides are sprayed on wheat and vegetable crops in the United States each year. That equals five pounds of toxins per person. According to experts, only 2 percent of these pesticides serve to protect the crops while the elements around the area absorb the rest of the chemicals. In most cities in America, water contains over seven hundred chemicals while ten thousand different chemicals used in food processing (Dr. Helena Toth Hardy, ND, CNC). Check it out yourself. I remember when we picked apples on Daddy Dewey's farm in Austin, Texas, who never let us throw an apple away that had a worm in it.

"If it didn't kill that worm, it won't kill us," he proclaimed. I haven't seen a worm in an apple in sixty years. My apples in my orchard had a few worms, but they didn't eat much. I treated my orchard with natural herbicides that are perfectly safe to all, including some of the worms. It did, however, also take care of the leaf mold. I don't get sick.

What about all those fruits and veggies imported from Chile, Mexico, and other parts of the world? Some of these countries are still using DDT, which was banned in our country decades ago. Do you realize that laws affecting the use of pesticides were created decades ago, and they have not been upgraded for years? All those laws were developed using a healthy adult male to set the standard for evaluation of the pesticides – not children, older folks, or the disable. It is ethically unacceptable that our children with their acutely sensitive nervous systems are being denied with basic protections by those antiquated laws that now exist. Why do I bring this important issue to your attention? Did you know right now in our country there is no process for reporting or monitoring adverse effects of pesticides? There have been only a few studies done on revealing the consequences of these pesticides to our bodies. There is no government process for reporting or monitoring the universal adverse effects from these pesticides. Why have I now reviled this information to you? The answer is simple. In that most of my readers are going to continue to consume the corporate-grown foods sold in the marketplace, then you have to consider applying a serious program for the detoxifying your body. These toxic chemicals are being stored in your body and represented a major threat to your life.

One contaminated apple may not kill you, but with the accumulation of a bushel or two over a period of time, you can bet your bottom dollar, your body is gathering, compounding, and storing toxins that will push your body to an early checking out from this planet. That, folks, is called toxic overloading; our immunity is negated, and slowly the disease will terminate our life. Maybe not tomorrow or next year, but you can be assured as Mother Nature made little green apples, your life will be terminated. As you should know, most of the people in this world die from the toxic overloading of their bodies; and that problem is a manmade and can be overcome, so read on.

One other thing that should be addressed is the taxpayer-funded subsidies that promote the farmers to use pesticides for crop protection. All toxic pesticides should be carefully reviewed, monitored, and studied under strict conditions at all times. Food producers should be constantly monitored by government to see that the laws controlling their use of pesticides is strictly enforced. Environmental agencies should be on the frontlines of keeping our food source safe and free from lethal chemicals that are polluting our planet as well as our bodies. All in all, we use tons of pesticides on our foods to deter bugs and enhance the cosmetic effect of the plant. This should be stopped immediately, and all pesticides used should be labeled on the fruits and vegetables. All federal laws and regulations that encourage the use of pesticides should be eliminated. Finally, no pesticides should be allowed to be used if there is an alternative natural pesticide that could be used that is safe and effective.

Where are those environmental quacks that are out there saving bugs and endangered worms and ignoring the endangered *Homo sapiens*? These outdated laws governing the use of pesticides in this country should be thrown out and brought up into the twentieth century. That cost should not be on the backs of the taxpayers, but the manufacturers.

One of your body's natural functions is to store what excess foods and nutrients you have eaten to be used at a later date. It has no idea or function for what to do with some of the toxins that accompany that food you eat. Your body has complete confidence in your ability and desire to choose the natural-grown foods that it requires to sustain your life. Unfortunately, your body has little or no control over what you eat – that's your mind – so it has to accept what you feed it. It has to adjust and be contented to live with confidence in your judgment to choose life-giving nutrients for it to consume. It just doesn't believe you will, in your right mind, feed it destructive poisons or foreign chemicals that it certainly can find no use for. It prefers to be ever trusting in your sound judgment and will store everything it can't find an immediate use for. I'm having breakfast at ten o'clock while I work; and it's a bowl of multigrains, bananas, blueberries, and soy milk. That will carry me over till my last meal for today which is around four o'clock. As we get older and less active, we should cut back on our food consumption. Every body is different, and you should monitor your daily consumption of food. Watch and record your energy levels against what you eat. It is a random study of your body's reaction to the foods you eat. Keep a simple chart of what you eat during the day and access your energy level.

Next, storing toxins is a very difficult and painful process for the body as they are all totally foreign particles; and if allowed to roam wild around the body, they would cause terminal damage to our organs or our life. Therefore, the body naturally provides a protective cover over the toxins, and now we could have a full-blown tumor in the making. Cancer is a deficiency and an autointoxication disease that is instigated by the overload of toxins in our bodies. The excess of toxins in our bodies causes toxicity that destroys good cells or transforms them into wild growing cells. We can summarize this statement by saying that we cause cancer cells to form in our bodies by what we eat and how we are able to process the foods we do eat. More detail later on this issue.

Regular exercising of the body is nature's natural means of cleansing and detoxifying the body through sweat and elimination tracts. As we exercise the body, we generate the loss of fluids in our body that carry out the important function of elimination of toxins. When we no longer keep the body tuned up and allow fatty, toxic globules to accumulate, we soon find our lives in deep trouble. I have a swivel chair at my computer, and it moves in many directions. My wife thinks I'm nuts when I go into contortions and do my exercises on my wobbly chair. This is a great invention for the whole body, and you just sit on it and wobble. More later if I take the time. The body, as we slow down, becomes overloaded with excess foreign matter; our energy levels drop; and our immune systems become stretched out with the constant struggle in protecting our lives. We can do better than that by setting a routine workout schedule.

The creation of these complex problems that stress out the natural life functions of our bodies is the primary cause of the body going berserk and developing all types of abnormal symptoms that may have nothing to do with the real problem. Pain suddenly develops in weird places, and when we go to the doctors about the pain, they say there's nothing wrong with you taking a pill. The body is experiencing something it is not quite sure how to deal with, but is sending out signals to you that something is wrong. Toxemia, which you don't hear much about in the medical field as it is the primary cause of most organ failures and can only be cured through natural means. The focus of the medical industry is on mysterious cancer-causing bugs; but the real underlying problem is toxemia, which is shutting the body's functions down, depleting energy, overloading immune system, and causing metabolic destruction.

There are many proven methods developed by the natural health industry to relieve your body from the effects of accumulative forms of toxemia. By following a well-documented cleansing program on a daily basis, we will free up our natural defenses that protect us from the effects of toxic buildup. This allows our body's immune systems to function as they were designed to – fighting bacteria and parasites that are consuming a big part of our life-giving nourishments. They are also the main contributors of the toxicity in our blood and organs as they deposit their waste in our bodies, and some are able to totally recycle their lives in our bodies. Now your life is in real, serious danger as it doesn't take long for that combination to totally saturate your body with toxins. We will deal with parasite critters later on.

Now, more *about radiation?* I am not going continue to beat a dead horse on this subject, but you should spend some more time educating yourself on this matter. I suggest you read the Web page at "Food Radiation: Who Is Killing Who?" The FDA has allowed radiated food to be sold to the public since 1963 without so much as a discloser label. Food must be safe if the FDA says so, right? Not always true. We should have confidence in the food we eat and enjoy knowing that we are getting the needed nourishment to sustain the life in our bodies. We should be free of worry and concern about our health. Life should be an experience of bliss and enjoyment, confident in having all the health needed to carry on normal daily functions. Are you confident that you are getting the needed nutrients and nourishment needed for your body's functions? Are there toxins and waste materials being stored in your body? I can answer that for you. If you're not watching what you are eating and not cleansing your body of toxic materials on a regular program, then you are a prime candidate for a toxic breakdown of your vital life functions. You may think I'm in left field, but after you read this material and you can still say that, I'll refund your cost of this book and listen to your rebuttal on why I'm off base in this issue. You see, if I don't address this important issue with all the honesty and openness I can express, I would be doing you, my readers, a gross injustice. Truth has many viewers with many conceptions and viewpoints. I'm confident, after reading this information, you will want to know what can be done to neutralize the damage that's being done with food that has been nuked with ten thousand or more radiation units.

Do you realize that with radiated food, we are introducing into our bodies foreign chemicals and toxic elements that are not found anywhere else on this planet. This is a major concern for the enlightened as many naturopaths are rightfully trying to address the problems as it is being brushed under the rug by the corporate government and totally ignored by the media. Do you ever question if our highly paid public servants who vote themselves pay raises in a faltering economy are really concerned over the welfare of the citizens of this nation? Politicians who are mostly programmed lawyers have had their interests and loyalties bought and paid for by special interest groups. They have sold out our nation's health interests to the drug cartel. Just look at the diminishing health of our society. Disease is running rampant all over the world. Did you ever believe you would have to live in fear of your government and be a witness to such a gross travesties being committed against their populations? Most of us who are concerned with the ongoing war for control of this planet know it will get worse before it gets better, but now is the time to take control of your life and its health activities.

Do you realize that it is high time for us to understand the full effects of all the potential poisons that we are taking into our bodies with the foods we eat? Most people are totally oblivious of this danger and don't really care as they have been programmed to have total confidence in the government's abilities to protect the welfare of its people. That's like having the fox look after the hen house. There are a few informed health patriots in our society that do care and know what's going on within the food industry and behind our backs.

Did you ever stop and wonder why there is an organically grown produce department in most grocery stores? Why is it more expensive to grow veggies naturally than to have them saturated with toxic chemicals? Wonder why there are naturally grown organic foods available at the grocery and health stores known also as Kosher foods. Also, very interesting is that they are expensive, and the normal buyer doesn't see the need to spend that extra money to buy them. Organically grown foods is only a small part of their business at those stores, and you probably wonder why they would bother carrying such small quantities of products for such a small group of clients. Only a handful of informed people who know something that we don't buy those products. I have never seen anyone looking at them, much less buy them. It seems logical to me if you are not spraying chemicals on those plants to keep the bugs off, then the products should be cheaper. Those selected buyers from their actions obviously know something the average grocery shopper doesn't. Give that some thought.

We now know that the grocery shelves are saturated with radiated, preserved foods that have harmful chemicals that are more dangerous than we realize. I would like for you to examine another Web page that has documented data that will give you a complete picture of the extent that our food has been radiated and what they are not telling you: naturalrearing.com and lifereasearchuniversal.com. This is a prime example of how corporate America manipulates its money powers into buying and controlling of government agencies. I always thought that government agencies were developed and created for the protection and preservation of the people.

Don't we pay their salaries? I guess we are not paying them enough to earn their loyalty and concern for our welfare. Maybe there is something in this movement to stop special interest groups from buying the loyalties of our politicos. Wonder why the masses don't raise up in anger and defiance over the injustice being dished out by the elected of our governments? We are all aware of the power and corruption being dealt to our nation by the corporate moguls. Could it be that over 70 percent of our population owns stock in corporate America? Read this Web page (All-organic-food.com) and become one of the few newly enlightened souls that are now avoiding dead, radiated foods and are enjoying the benefits of wholesome, homegrown, natural foods.

Again, as a born-again, ham actor, I enjoy keeping things visual; so we will attack our health problems with vigor, anger, and decisive action. We also need to see the progress we make. We should set up a regular weekly program for eliminating toxins from our bodies. That starts with drinking plenty of pure water, not Coca-Cola. Drinking coffee, sodas, and alcohol actually dehydrates the body – read *Your Body's Many Cries for Water*. It is recommended by many naturopaths that we drink eight- to ten-ounce glass of water a day. As we have reiterated, the body becomes overburdened with junk waste products and – without the flushing process of pure water, which doing without – prevents trillions of our cells from being nourished properly from the food we eat.

First place to start is in our toxic cleanup program with drinking water that makes up over 70 percent of our body's material.

The colons, large and small, are the passageway for all the nourishment you get from the foods that you eat. You can't let it get clogged up with decaying, putrefied foods that just sit there, rotting away in your body. Many people have been known to carry in the access of thirty pounds of dead, fecal matter just rotting away in their intestinal tracts. Ask any colonic practitioner who perform colon cleanses on hundreds of people yearly (Global Institute for Alternative Medicine). You just have to look at the potbellies running around our society to know something is wrong. This sight will have some added information as a clogged colon is a gigantic problem in our society today and needs to be addressed seriously by anyone that is going to consider having and maintaining optimum health. We need to know how to totally wash out our colons and keep them clean in order for them to operate at top performance. That not only means fasting on a regular basis but using plenty of water that does not allow the putrefied and decayed fecal matter to clog up in our intestinal tracts. Water, not chlorinated but pure, will aid in keeping the colon flushed out while the natural enzymes and digestive juices are doing their job of nourishing every cell in our body. However, if you already have a real health problem with overweight and toxicity, then you need to seriously consider a more effective, rigorous means of cleansing the gut. To take control of this problem starts with colon cleanses with taking periodic coffee enemas. This method of cleansing the colon once or more times a week is totally dependent on your assessment of your personal health. How much energy are you receiving from the food you eat?

How well do you really feel about your general health? Only you can truthfully determine this factor. If you're lethargic and tired all the time, constipated and have a hard time being regular in you bowel movements, then your body is definitely showing undue stress and not functioning up to par. How toxic is your body? That is hard to determine as illness always moves slowly in overloading and stressing out your whole system. It's hard to determine your health status as the disease process creeps up on us gradually. What you have to do is read the indicators such as we start by passing stinky gas, intestinal bloating, aches, pains, and general ill feelings. Final test is the lack of energy, and depression sets in. We are prone to go to the over-the-counter drugs, drinking juices, and local general practitioners for relief, looking for quick fix to a long-time-developing problem. Be sure and read carefully all the side affects from the drugs the doctor prescribes for your symptoms. Do you have any idea how many folks are living on drug care? Let me give you a few enlightening statistics. The prestigious Institute of Medicine yielded some chilling fact: "Adverse reactions to medications kills 108,000 people each year." Now mind you, the drug-related deaths are not from overdoses or misuse of prescription drugs, they represent individuals taking prescription drugs under a doctor's supervision and in accordance with the manufacturer's protocols. Altogether this means that some 227,000 people die each year from deficiencies in hospitals and prescription drugs! To put the figure in perspective, that's 4.3 times as many patients died from doctor's incompetence than during the ten years of the Vietnam War!

This information was printed in the *Journal of the American Medical Association* in July 26, 2000.

Even if that doesn't move you, maybe this will. We, the victims of the medical corporation giants, spend trillions on health care benefits and lead the entire world in that category; but we are the world's sickest society with over half our society having some form of chronic illness. We are the most overweight, undernourished population on this planet. Does that sound like some kind of conspiracy or not? Are you eating to stay alive or to please your taste buds. Are you eating the proper kinds of foods in their natural state? Look, if your energy is zapped out, you feel stuffed and needed to lie down to rest after eating; then you have given way to gluttony. The older you become, the less you need to eat as your metabolism has slowed down, and your energy levels are lowered. It is high time you concern yourself with eating proper foods. Why eat to just pacify your taste buds and fill your gut? Eat less and meet the needs of the body, not the taste buds. Feel that fat circle around your waist. That's the extra scoop of ice cream, cake, or another sweet cookie that you have become accustomed to eating after a big meal. Did you know that some people carry in excess of thirty pounds of stagnate fecal matter just sitting and rotting in their intestinal tract? The only function for your intestinal tract is the digesting of all foods it's given and turn it into life-giving enzymes and minerals to nourish and feed the millions of cells in your body. This process is greatly hampered and impaired when the bulk of the food you eat is useless, preprocessed, and foreign to the body garbage that has to be eliminated.

The ideal situation is the body receives wholesome, natural foods, dripping with enzymes, vitamins, and fibers where the digestive process becomes fast and simple. Food is broken down into enzymes, and vital elements are then distributed in the blood to nourish every cell in our bodies. Blood doesn't normally carry waste material into the body; however, when the body becomes overloaded and saturated with toxins, then it is given with no other choice. Your body reacts to the poisons you have fed it by trying desperately to rid the body of the poisons through the skin or any other means; it has to protect the life of your organs. Can you see it is your first priority and imperative to your health that your intestinal track functions properly with optimum efficiency? Having a clean and functional intestinal tract that eliminates all waste materials with two to three daily bowel movements will add years to your life expectancy and grant you a head start on obtaining and maintaining optimum health. Do I have your attention?

Added to this program, if possible, is the taking of steam baths or saunas once a week. This process needs close monitoring as it depends on how toxic your body has become and the amount of fat your have accumulated. Our skin is a vital organ in ridding of toxins and fats that accumulate under the skin. I try to take Jacuzzis on a weekly schedule as they are very relaxing and assist the body in its task of ridding the unwanted foreign materials while reducing fat and excess liquids in the body. I put two cups of Epson salts and one cup of apple vinegar in my bath to soak in along with small bottle of peroxide 3 percent. This is very beneficial in killing parasites and drawing toxins out of our systems.

Remember, folks, our goal is going after all the excessive waste products that have accumulated and stored throughout the parts of the body. We know there is no area in our body that is not a target to our detoxifying process as the parasites and toxins have been well distributed throughout our bodies. To get healthy, you must enjoy having the full benefit of the food you eat. If your digestive process is plagued with deteriorating garbage that's blocking and stressing out its natural functions, then it's time you get the system reamed out and flowing naturally.

There are a multitude of herbs on the market that claim colon-cleansing properties. You should consult with your naturopath if you have cramps and bloating and irregularity in elimination. You need to find some program that works for you and use it religiously, particularly if you are going to continue consuming a lot of that great-tasting junk food. Regular stools are mandatory for health, so it is imperative to get your body on a regular schedule – twice a day is the least to expect (healingdaily.com).

When you physically take over the responsibility of cleansing your body of toxins, parasites, and excess fat modules, you are liberating your immune system from a lot of stress so that it can remain focused on all those foreign critters that are trying to take over your body. Keep your body alive and kicking from the miry attacks of parasites, viruses, and other diseases that we are exposed to in this present polluted planet. Do you now understand why the main threat to our lives is the plague of toxemia? If our bodies are liberated from the effects of septicemia, microorganism in the blood, we are on that path to optimum health.

I want to support my position by quoting Stanley Burroughs, *The Master Cleanser*, who made popular the lemonade diet.

> Disease, old age, and death are the result of accumulated poisons and congestions throughout the body. These toxins become crystallized and hardened, settling around the joints, in the muscles, and throughout the billions of cells all over the body. It is presumed by orthodox medicine that we have a perfectly healthy body until something, such as germs or viruses, come along to destroy it, such as actually the building material for the organs and cells is defective, and thus, they are inferior or diseased. Lumps and growths are formed all over the body as storage spots *for unusable and accumulated waste products*, especially in the lymphatic glands. These accumulations depress and deteriorate in varied degrees, causing degeneration and decay. The liver, spleen, colon, stomach, heart, and our other organs, glands, and cells come in for their share of accumulations, thus, impairing their natural action.

> These growths and lumps appear to us as forms of fungi. *Their spread and growth is dependent on the unusable waste and toxic material throughout the body.* As deterioration of body functions continues, our growth lumps increases in size to take care of the growing situation. Fungi absorb the poisons and toxins that want to attack and destroy our organs. This is part of nature's plan to rid the body of our diseases. When

we stop feeding this fungi, cleanse our systems, we stop their development and spreading. They can then dissolve into the bloodstream and pass out from the body.

They cannot feed on healthy tissue. There is a simple set of laws which explains this action. Nature never produces anything it does not need, and it never keeps anything it does not use. All unused material or waste is broken down by bacteria action into a form that can be used later or eliminated from the body. All weak and deficient cells, caused from improper nutrition, will also be broken down and eliminated from the body. We spend a good portion of our lives accumulating these diseases, and we spend the rest of our lives attempting to get rid of them or die in the effort.

The incorrect understanding of the above truths has led uncivilized nations alike to search for some magic "cure" in all kinds of charms, witchcraft, and unlimited kinds of obnoxious poisons and drugs. In general, they are worse than useless because they cannot possibly eliminate the poisons and drugs. They can only add more misery and suffering and shorten one's life still further. It has been reported in many books and magazine articles that many new diseases and disorders have been created by orthodox and hospital methods. As we continue to search for more and more magic cures, we become more and more involved with complicated varieties of diseases. Understanding, along with positive actions, have always proven to be the best means to eliminate our negative actions and reactions. "Germs and viruses do not and cannot cause any of our diseases, so we have no need for finding various kinds of poisons to destroy them. In fact, man will never find a poison or group of poison strong enough to destroy all the billions of billions of these germs without destroying himself at the same time.

These germs are our friends, there are no bad ones and, if given a chance, will break up and consume these large amounts of waste matter and assist us in eliminating them from the body. These germs and viruses exist in excess only when we provide a breeding ground in which they can multiply. Germs and viruses are in the body to help break down waste material and can do no harm to healthy tissues.

We know that throughout nature everything moves in cycles, constantly changing, constantly cleaning out the old and rebuilding the new. Consequently, as a person reaches the "point of no return," a point where his accumulations have reached the limit of what the body can tolerate, then rapid change takes place or he dies. The cycle has come to the point where good house cleaning must be started and one of nature's most effective methods is to start loosening and eliminating these poisons with bacteria action. As this action progresses, we come sick and feverish, large amounts of mucus are eliminated, diarrhea increases the discharge of waste material, and all of our resources go into action to clean us out as fast as possible to prevent these poisons from killing us. When this happens, do not panic and resort to the unnatural action of drugs and antibiotics, which can only defeat nature's laws. Most drugs we are given stop the natural changes by suppressing the cleansing action and store the poisons in the body to cause future problems.

Becoming toxic by not controlling the unfriendly parasites will deter your ability to free up energy necessary to support your immune system and maintain a fulfilling and productive life.

I can't emphasize the importance of doing an intensive study on the Internet and reading pertinent books on the complete process of toxic elimination that includes the maintenance of the intestinal tract. This is the most important key to optimum health. Without a proper cleansing program designed for *you* to meet your body's needs, your life can never be free from stress and discomfort caused by bacteria overload of your system. Your health program must incorporate an ongoing, complete cleansing of the body. We are living in a polluted world that supports a host to hundreds of species of living parasites that are being offered daily into our bodies for the development of new diseases, subnormal body functions, and untold types of physical disorders. New diseases are being discovered all over the world, which have become immune to antibiotics and our immune systems. You don't need to offer your bodies as feeding grounds for these little creatures. So now that I have opened Pandora's box, let's really examine these microscopic living organisms that have found a home in our bodies. Let's label this next paragraph the "silent killers." You are going to read information that is going to turn your attitude toward maintaining good health into a full-fledged war zone with your body being the battlefield. It is a real conflict that never ends, and we have accepted up front that our bodies are going to lose in the final analysis; however, as Bush would say, "Bring them *on!*" That could be morbid image of your future or a positive activity that you can claim victory over disease now and live a long, prosperous, disease-free life passing away in your sleep, dreaming of life in the presence of our Creator.

At seventy-eight, I can personally witness to the reality that we do have life after death. This body may terminate, but the soul finds peace and comfort within that is expressed in all that life functions. It is very difficult to find this inner peace without enjoying good health as we become focused and stressed out on the diseases that threatens our lives. When we enjoy the confidence of our good health status, our emotions and spirits are free to receive and obtain the spiritual assurance that confirms that our Creator coexists within our lives. Finding that divine peace within ourselves that passes all understanding, we are able to make progress on the ultimate purpose for our existence on this planet. God's divine purpose is unique and personal to all creation and yours to obtain and acknowledge.

Chapter 3

Our Unknown Killers

MANY DOCTORS ATTEST to the fact that parasites are affecting the health of eight out of ten Americans. I contend as well as many other experts in this field that all humans play host to hundreds of different varieties of microscopic parasites. Can you tell me why haven't the pharmaceutical moguls, who could reap millions of dollars on developing new drugs for disease, haven't developed one single drug to control the infestation of these microscopic living creatures? Is it *simply* because our little inhabitants are the second main contributors to all the disease and illnesses found plaguing the world societies? Their little life cycle of living and slowly eating away at our body fluids has developed a very lucrative business that underwrites the multimillion-dollar industries of drug cartels and medical professions.

The pharmaceutical industry alone made 182 billion dollars in drug sales last year. I would not even venture a guess on how much the medical profession brought to the table.

Controlling the world's parasite infestations would alter the toxic buildup in humanity and dig heavily into the profits of the international drug and medical industries. It is sad that all the monies we have donated to the researching of new drugs with all their side effects has gone to develop just treatments for all the various diseases (no cures). None of that money has been spent on pursuing methods to control and possibly rid the body of one of the main underlying causes for disease – parasitic infestation.

We will have to dig into the natural health field to find natural proven means to effectively control and eliminate those little microscopic critters that inhabit our bodies. Stop and consider that something so small you can't see is living off your body's nourishments. Your immune system is constantly at work neutralizing their devastating effects on your life force. That is the primary job of white blood cells. It actually zaps them out with an electrical charge.

"The single most undiagnosed health challenge in the history of the human race is parasites. I realize that is a pretty brave statement, but it is based on my twenty years of experience with more than twenty thousand patients," said Dr. Ross Anderson, ND. "We have a tremendous parasite problem right here in the United States. It is just not being addressed," said Dr. Peter Wina of Walter Reed Hospital. "In terms of numbers, there are more parasitic infections acquired in this country than in Africa," said Dr. Frank Nova, chief for the Laboratory for Parasitic Diseases for the National Institute of Health.

We will now address the methodology of controlling our aggressive parasitic inhabitants that maintain a constant threat to our health and lives. Just look for a moment at all the money that's gathered in the name of nonprofit organizations, looking for a cure for every deadly disease known to man. How many millions of grant dollars have been wasted on scams, promoting research and studies that goes nowhere as they intentionally ignore the culprit behind most diseases in our bodies, the parasite? We are losing the battle against viruses and bacteria. The antibiotics are being rendered ineffective as the bugs have become resistant to most of the pharmaceutical drugs. There is no amount of research, time, or money that will perfect a cure for any diseases until you recognize, accept, and treat the primary cause. Our micro-controlled medical system has no intention of finding the cures for anything as long as their victims are willing to pay and accept the temporary treatments that suppress the symptoms. The simple, natural cures presented in this little book, as recorded by the best natural health servants on this planet, could totally disrupt the world medical system. It would create economic instability in the medical field, putting millions of medical personnel into other professions. You can bet this book will not be on a best seller's list, but I will probably have to present my findings to a few curious souls that might buy this e-book on my Web site. "Truth must have an avenue to travel and a following to keep it alive." Truth is the only force that can combat the ignorance of greed and power that possess the lives of the world managers. All rational, thinking men and women know that truth will ultimately win out.

The proven truths we establish for our lives during this temporal existence on this planet are the only foundation that makes mankind's journey on this planet tolerable. I started researching this book five years ago using my body as a proving ground for the technology I have uncovered in the natural health industry. We are nearing an abyss right now with greed and fear in control of man's future. I am seventy-eight going on one hundred, living with no fear of some incurable disease killing me.

There exists in this world knowledge of cures for all diseases. That's a truth you must first desire to believe, and then you can seek its manifestation and evidence in your life. Upon your accepting and believing that statement, your health becomes a part of your belief system that you can bring into reality. The first vital step is *belief, which brings us into a positive profile that will reap benefits. The most difficult part of dealing with disease is to put your life on a positive footing.* Our minds and lives have been programmed to rely on the flawed billion-dollar medical system and its massive resources and gimmicks to treat and solve all our health problems. Remember, doctors are not by accident the third largest contributors of deaths in our society – more than traffic accidents and gun accidents put together. They have a place in our society, but our lives and health remain our personal responsibility. We should never allocate that responsibility into a flawed health system that has the reputation that our medical system has racked up. It is another money-orientated system that reaps millions in monetary gains while millions die at their hands. Remember, certain God-given freedoms should always be respected.

We have been given by our Creator certain inalienable rights, and number one is the right to make those life-affecting decisions that pertain to our personal health. What is lacking in this picture is having total access to all information on alternative methods and cures being developed in the naturopathic and homeopathic health industries. That coveted information properly exposed will assist all of us in making those lifesaving, informed decisions needed to preserve our lives. Our political servants should assure and demand that we the people have access to the best health information available in the marketplace. After you have been offered the evidence from all sides of the picture, then the final decision rests in your corner. Today's health services in the curing marketplace are primary one-sided allopathic. I am totally convinced that the vital information on hundreds of natural health remedies for our nation's terminal sick will never come from the conventional drug system. So therefore, you are going to be confronted now with a presentation of many natural cures that I will not try to convince you to accept or reject but will just present facts and findings. The private and personal testimonies of the patients that have all been affected by the applications of natural remedies will be all evidence presented that you will have to make your decisions on. The natural health industry will challenge you to accept their methods of cures based on extensive studies, empirical knowledge, and personal testimonies of the many souls that have been cured by applying their natural remedies. They have – through biology, chemistry, and human testing – determined and proven the effects of their treatments.

Many are based on cures and remedies that have been developed and passed down from many world social systems like Japan, China, Africa, etc. The Internet has given me and my support group access to all the unconventional natural methods of treating all forms of disease worldwide. I call this world movement to expose to the world the natural cures God created for mankind the Underground Natural Health Movement (UN-HeM).

The more effective and exposed these natural cures have become in our society, the more aggressive the medical institutions become in suppressing the information. The medical profession has its own group of highly paid police forces just to prevent the natural health industry from exposing and promoting inexpensive, effective, and proven natural health remedies. Many a fine, informed, and respectable natural health practitioners has been defamed, fined, looted, threatened, and even incarcerated by the stooges of the medical institutions. They know well that the allopathic drug industry, with its renowned record of not curing anyone, are no real competition or threat to the competent and dedicated group of natural biologists and scientists who are freethinkers and altruistically motivated. They have the welfare and concern for the human race as number one priority. They will risk life and limb to bring you the truths and cures to aid the world populations in obtaining the natural health remedies that God intended man to experience and enjoy.

Our medical professionals, along with the governmentally protected drug industries, have a complete different approach to illness. They never assume there is a medical cure for any disease.

Their approach to man's diseases is they have treatments as the means to treat patients. Being a doctor is a prestigious position in our society that is revered and envied. He is no longer a servant to mankind but an icon. The term *doctor* automatically elevates that schooled person into privileged class. Doctors are taught to treat the systems which they can determine from the information you give them along with a few expensive tests. Now, they make an educated prognosis and guess to determine a treatment for your illnesses and then prescribe the appropriate drugs that hopefully will suppress the systems and give your body the opportunity to cure yourself. Doctors do not cure patients; the body does. They may aid in some ways, but patients cure patients, and that's what we are all about.

The data and documentation in this book is only knowledge, a guideline to assist you in making alternative health decisions for yourself. We will uncover vital truths that have been purposely suppressed from the mainstream news media. We will expose you to proven natural cures that you can have confidence and assurance that they will support the body's functions to affect a cure. It will be your decision as to the source and creditability of the medical information before you ever considered it for an application into your life. My position in this endeavor is to point you to the verse and scriptures and leave you to have the responsibility to determine for yourself if it's applicable to your symptoms. Many of the cures are trial and error as all bodies are uniquely different and diagnosis will vary as do the symptoms and amount of contamination. Remember, it's a natural product, not some synthetic, toxic drug that you are consuming.

It is you and your natural instincts that is determining factor in the severity of the illness affecting your body. Sometimes, we have various illnesses that give off different signals, and we attempt to address those issues. We can become confused in our self-diagnosis process; however, if we remain persistent and learn the symptoms from our experiences, we will start diagnosing what ails us from the symptoms being given off.

The key is being in tune with your body. Listen to it as it speaks to you. Know that it always has needed for vital nourishment. Know that when it develops a condition of illness that it didn't happen overnight, so the cure won't come overnight. As you question and then determine for yourself the nature of the problem, remember to look for the cause. Start your cure with eliminating the cause, then perfect a cure, and monitor your recovery. When dealing with natural products, you may not put your life in jeopardy, but it certainly doesn't mean that everything you take will affect a cure overnight. Our cures are a form of belief system based on intelligent and documented information we find or experience. Is it foolproof? Will it cure all my problems? Of course not. Only your body can do that, but you will give your body every opportunity available to rejuvenate itself naturally. The natural approach to health care is opening the means for you to regain optimum health by natural means without having to deal with toxic drugs. The real evidence of your self-curing process will only appear as the body reacts to the natural assistance you give it. The body does the work on you, give it the tools to perfect its natural function of self-preservation. Drink plenty of water to continue to flush toxins out of the body.

Curing the body starts with curing the mind of depression, negativity, and despondent thoughts. Control your thoughts, and believe in yourself and the choices that you make. They will be made on best available information that you can search the Internet and in health books. Trust your instincts that good physical results will soon appear as you apply daily applications of proven health practices. We can make changes in our lives when we have the confidence in the choices we made that are necessary and founded on sound principles and documentation. We also must have confidence in the intent of the messenger. My influence in this vital matter stops here with this book. You're on your own after you read the information that I have collected for you. I have only one request if you find my observations not trustworthy or valid, please contact me at my Web page and give me all your assessments and disagreements. I am certainly not infallible like doctors, and I believe deeply in being flexible. I've made a few mistakes in my life to say the least and will probably make a few more before I cash in.

Now let's hit the quasi-medical establishment another way. You can go on supporting the myriad of different so-called nonprofit organizations that are advertising in media, promoting an endless search for cures for various deadly diseases that kill millions of our citizens each year. Those bleeding hearts have been raping and pilfering the public for years and will never perfect a cure as it is not profitable. If they found the cure, they would be out of business. The medical industry would go broke if God's natural cures were perfected and publicized.

What really makes sense out of all this and holds true is *if you can catch it, you can cure it.* Alzheimer, common colds, AIDS, SARS, cancer, you name it – we are prime targets for the world scam artists that live off the sick and dying. The list of incurables will always exist in the media as it produces an attitude of despondency and hopelessness that leads to panic and desperate actions. The saturation of their drug promotion in the media is vital in reaching the masses to propagate and establish creditability to their drug-producing industry. Do you realize that hundreds of drugs are out there would be deemed useless if natural cures were perfected and marketed as the synthetics are not without side effects? New diseases are cropping up all the time, and you can bet your bottom dollar that the pharmacies are right behind with a drug treatment. "Have you tried the purple pill? Ask you doctor it the purple pill is right for you." It's almost like clockwork. Once a week, we hear of a new virus; and a few weeks later, we have a drug treatment. Could it be they were developed at the same time?

The drug companies have spent millions to suppress all the natural cures that have been developed by mankind since the beginning of time. If those same natural cures were being investigated, developed, and perfected on the same scale as synthetic drugs, can you imagine the impact it would make on the condition of the health of our nation? Are the people in our nation truly free? If we were truly free, wouldn't we have access to all the technology and natural cures afforded the rich and famous? The elite are working on the means to live forever; and I wonder if we, the not-so privileged, will be privy to that knowledge.

Have you heard that we are real close to a cancer cure? We have been for years, and the donations keep flowing in. Well, I got news for you, a cure has been perfected and is being used by many doctors in other parts of the world. That's why the wealthy go to Europe or Mexico. The media hype with their pathetic advertisements will keep the donations coming in, and hope is alive without helping the afflicted and the dying. Can you think of a better scam to strip a dying cancer patient out of his last shekels before you bury him? We all know they are always making tremendous progress, and a cure will be perfected next year or maybe the next. Millions die every year needlessly of cancer with absolutely no hope or help from our medical system. You'll like this new approach? Hundreds, diagnosed with a fatal disease, are being frozen in vaults with the hope and belief that there will be a cure perfected someday; and then they can be revived and enjoy the rest of their natural life with good health. It takes a real creative person to think of the ways to rip off the sick and the dying. Do I sound a little bitter?

My first reaction to the documentation that parasites are living in my body was sort of like my wife's "Please leave me alone, I don't want to hear about parasites infecting my body. I can't see them; besides, we don't live in a third world country, and we are one of the most sterile and highly developed societies in the world." To this day, she doesn't want to discuss the little creatures living inside her body; but she does recognize they are there, and she keeps her preventive program going on a weekly basis as I do. At seventy-eight, my immune system needs all the support I can give it; and believe me, I don't let it down.

Now we are going to elaborate on the topic of infestation of parasites living in and off our body's fluids. We will explore exactly what effect they have on our health, both good and bad. We must expose all the potential dangers that this unseen living organism can create in our bodies. I just read that the globalists' forces in our world are working to harness and develop this living, deadly organism to bring about a selective world culling of populations through DNA selectivity. I will not address this issue as it is only computer hearsay, but I will address the methods and means to keep these parasites under control and how to protect your life from being subject to biochemical destruction that is a real threat to our world today.

We are going to learn how to deal with the symptoms and results of their lives being recycled within our bodies. Let's quote another well-known author and nutritionist, Ann Louis Gittleman, "You may be an unsuspecting victim of the parasite epidemic that is affecting millions of Americans. It is an epidemic that knows no territorial, economic, or sexual boundaries. It is a silent epidemic of which most doctors in this country are not even aware." Now here is another. "A parasite is an organism that lives off the host, the host being you or me. The parasite lives in a parallel life inside our bodies, feeding off, either our own energy, our own cells, or the food we eat. Parasites are even feeding off the health supplements we use, thus, greatly diminishing their effectiveness," said Dr. Ross Anderson, one of the foremost parasitic infection specialists in America. Remember, it's not the intention of the parasites to kill its victims; they just live off it. Many of those buggers are beneficial to our existence.

The life-threatening process only comes into prominence when the body is overloaded with parasitic toxicity and the body's nourishment is all used to nourish the billions of parasites that it's now supporting. The outcome is infestation of the body's organs, resulting in failure and toxicity. The body's immune systems can only handle certain amount of toxicity before the organs become stressed out and start to shut down. We virtually reach a point where every normal function of the body goes in to stress, confusion, and dysfunction. Our bodies virtually go into a form of walking shock with the death march playing in the background. It's a morbid picture that's being played out continuously all around us. This once-free nation of freethinking souls is now a massive disaster area waiting to collapse in chronic sickness and mental desperation.

My daughter-in-law is a nurse, and she has witnessed hundreds of deaths due to the ignorance and incompetence of well-meaning doctors who have never been taught how to cure diseases, but only to treat them. Go while you can and purchase at your health food store *The Cure for All Disease* by Dr. Hulda Clark. She has other books that are even more informative, but get this book first as it is a must in your pursuit of optimum health. I bought mine at my local health food store, but I am informed that the medical cartel are trying desperately to get her books off the shelves and put her in prison. This one book has opened my eyes to the path of enjoyable living. It has performed miracles in changing my lifestyle, and she truly has become my personal guru. She is not just a fine and saintly soul, but she has a great calling on her life that has already helped millions all over the world.

She is a saintly knight standing alone against the drug-controlled medical system. She has stood the test of time and given her life to the protection our right to have access to vital information on natural cures for all diseases. She has single-handedly fought the medical cartel for our right to have access to scientific data that will protect the lives of the laymen in our society against the misconception that only college-trained doctors with a degree from an accredited medical institute can practice medicine. She single-handedly has restored our God-given right to have access to information and products that are proven to sustain life and cure disease. She is a biochemist who once worked for the U.S. government. She has fought those medical monopolies in the courts all over our land and in Europe. She has that German tenacity and a dedication to help the helpless. God truly has protected her as they have made every attempt possible to discredit and nullify her influence in the health industry. It has been my observation that when some gallant brave soul is persecuted by the medical system for their contribution to the health of our society, it is because their information is valid and the products defined work as proclaimed. It's obvious that all natural cures that can't be bought or patented threatens the massive drug industry that has a stronghold on the health of the world. Believe me, the whole force of the medical cartel is out to get her books off the shelves of the health food stores nationwide, so get them while you can. Her Web page is dr.huldaclark.com is the best reading you can indulge in as it is the basic key to optimum health. It has been my total dedication to living a long and enriched life filled with God's love.

According to the Partnership for Solutions, led by Johns Hopkins University and the Robert Wood Johnson Foundation, more than 125 million Americans (half our population) have at least one chronic condition, and 60 million have more than one chronic condition. Examples of chronic conditions are cancer, heart disease, diabetes, and glaucoma. Are you one of the complacent Americans who's willing to accept being one of those statistics? Is your personal health not really important until it's threatened with death? I stopped by on my way back from the film festival in Lone Pine, California, to see an old actor friend I had worked with many times over. He was having difficult time enjoying our visit due to his health condition. He died a few days later. It wasn't his death that really hit me as he was over eighty-three and had a great life. What really hit me was the way he was existing on the end of an oxygen bottle with a handful of pills and confined to his chair. Think again, seriously, if enjoying optimum health is not a major concern and goal for your life. The problem of parasites affecting your life is not going away, but is in fact increasing to where it is estimated to rise to 157 million people who will be infested in the year 2020, and medical cost will double to more than $1 trillion. Millions of our fellow citizens cannot afford health care insurance, and millions are forced to live without it. Now I hear the hospitals all over the nation are no longer being forced to care for the indigents or homeless. It's time we all look after ourselves and get big medical institutions out of our lives. I remember when government was just a small group of elected statesmen we sent to Washington to protect our nation's freedoms.

Not true today as we can no longer afford all the government agencies and career politicos have become our demise and rulers as they have submerged the Constitution in a meaningless rhetoric that has no force or effect. We now have government of elites who are career bureaucrats that control the affairs of the people from cradle to grave. The concept of "We the people" is a mockery to justice and truth as the established political career are there to control the affairs of this nation from cradle to grave. Politicians are career oriented to death as long as they don't rock the boat like Robert Kennedy.

We are now going to consider a killing program to rid and control those little microscopic varmints that are the number one cause of all the world's health problems. There are many natural methods of controlling parasites in our bodies as mankind has been fighting this problem since the beginning of time. Every society has developed its own natural methods of performing this task, and we will address some of the best of these customs. As you are now aware, we all take the critters to the grave with us as they will win the battle in the long run. That doesn't say we can't keep them under control and complete our high calling in Jesus Christ. That is a worthy cause and godly goal to complete. I'm confident that is within the divine plan that God has for all our lives. I have been on that path for years and spent much of that time undoing the damage I performed on my life in the forty-odd years I spent in the film industry. Hopefully, you don't have that problem to deal with, but I'm confident that most Americans are fast-food victims and neglectful to the damage they are doing to their lives.

Hopefully, after reading this repetitious, boring commentary, you will be willing to change your eating habits – and to eat food to nourish the body, not because of the taste buds. Having started with some alterations in your life and common old horse sense, we are ready to attack the root cause of most of our health problems – *the food we eat.* This is going to be a tough row to hoe. We are addicted to the foods we consume and feel they have sustained our lives for all these years, why should I consider a cuisine adjustment? We are what we eat. If you are fighting the Battle of the Bulge, with which I have a film made in Spain, then start thinking seriously about a cuisine change. You start by changing some of the types of foods you eat and adjusting the portion you are consuming. This is a major giant step in regaining a good health and a must for you to sustain optimum health in your life. I can't emphasize the magnitude of the importance of eating properly vitalized food with restraint. There is nothing wrong with leaving the table with space enough for a second dessert. I don't mean to beat a dead horse, but if you are going to restore and stabilize your eating habits, start with the desserts. Nothing is alive and nourishing for the body in ice cream and cake. When you are not consuming live foods, then you are depriving your body and forcing it to digest garbage it has no use of. It needs nourishments to maintain and restore the vitality and energy you are expending every minute you live. All we do is expend energy in whatever we are doing. We only rest from that action when we are in a deep sleep, and the body shuts down. That is the time of restoring and building our life force that supports and nourishes all our vital organs.

Enough said for now as we will now focus our attention on methods of controlling our antagonists – the parasites. The methods I will introduce have proven successful to work for me and millions of others. As we said, there are many recorded methods of killing the critters in the archives of medicine archives. It has been at constant plague of mankind's existence since the beginning of time even before we could detect their presence in our bodies. Over the years, many natural methods of parasite control have been developed. All these natural remedies have been passed down from generation to generation by our ancestors, and we're all directed at controlling unfriendly parasites even though they were unable to see or determine how they caused the illnesses. What they were able to show is if they took certain herbs and tonics, they could curtail and treat their illnesses, thus allowing their bodies to perfect a cure. The information on these natural cures have been erased from our new age societies with a well-orchestrated master plan that used the controlled media, medical profession, and the drug companies with their powerful influence over the political hacks that have sold out our Republic to the globalists. Have you noticed how the drug cartel is presently going directly to the consumer with a constant barrage of TV proper gander, selling their synthetic drugs direct to the public? Today, it is a new way of life, and our society has no clue how to naturally combat or cure personal illnesses without the assistance of the medical cartel. Our forefathers would turn over in their graves if they could see the amount of synthetic drugs subjecting our bodies to find a use for. We are going back in time to reinvent natural cures.

We will start our program with a parasite control that has been proven to be the root cause of most diseases. One of the most effective means of killing off these unwanted parasites is a combination of herbs as directed by Dr. Hulda Clark in her book *The Cure for All Diseases.* There are three ingredients in her program, green black walnut hulls, wormwood, and cloves. I take this formula on an empty stomach in the morning for three days each month. Two teaspoons of the combination of wormwood and black walnut in a consecrate tincture product made by NOW found at your health food store. That can be taken by an empty stomach in the morning with an eight-ounce glass of ozonated water. With that, I take two gel caps of fresh cloves. I take this combination for three days every month just for maintenance. However, for the first-time person, the method is more intense. Check with her book for the complete program, and follow it to the letter. This is a woman who knows what she is talking about and has a following like no other natural healer on the planet.

Vibrantwellness.com is another Web site offering a sound cleansing program from the Mediterranean herbs that has been passed down for decades. Also worth mentioning is drnatura.com as it has a fine program for colon cleansing. Both are a bit pricey, *but* you get what you pay for; and when it comes to your health, don't be skimpy. I haven't tried the more complicated process of cleansing the intestine, but I am going to the next time I do the program again, which I do at least twice a year. Be totally convinced that this is one of the primary responsibilities you have in obtaining optimum health, so do it regularly, and get on with your life.

Remember 90 percent of all disease and discomfort is directly related to a parasite-infested colon that's impacted with fecal matter buildup. John Wayne was reported to have over twenty pounds of fecal matter in his colon at death. Now I am going to support my findings with another professional that has supported the use of the black walnut combination. He has a very good Web page that is worth reading (Wildernessfamilynaturals.com). I mean, to get you informed and convinced that this cleansing process of your colon is essential to achieving optimum health. After you have gone through the killing programs and then set up your personal control maintenance system to keep the no-see-um's under control, then and only then can you relax with the confidence that you are on your way to living a disease-free existence. Another Web page that supports an intense parasite cleansing of the body (parasite cleanse) is at seasilvertreadnet. com. The bottom line is to stop the mire of parasites from depositing their toxins in your blood systems. This program of cleansing your body from all alien forces from the environment is the ultimate process in maintaining and securing optimum health for your future on our planet. Note: Pesticides consumed by man from the food he eats do not affect the parasites in his body.

Last note: Almost 1.5 billion pounds of pesticides are sprayed on wheat and vegetables crops in the United States each year. That's more than five pounds per person yearly. The average American is exposed to fifty thousand chemical agents in his lifetime, and only a fraction of these have been studied for their effects on humans (Dr. Helena Toth Hardy, ND, CNC).

Many forms of parasites living in a toxic environment are now able to completely recycle all their reproduction capabilities within our bodies. You now are playing host to a family of bacteria that no longer have the need for other environments to reproduce its life cycle now. Bacteria are aerobatic in that they cannot live in the presence of oxygen. If they find themselves in an oxygen environment, they just leave the scene or hibernate till we make their lives more adaptable and comfortable with toxicity. Hopefully, at this time, you have realized the importance of cleaning up the environment of your body's system by keeping it clean.

One thing that I would like to bring out is a motivating experience I had some four years ago. I suddenly found that I could no longer control my bladder. I was having trouble going to the bathroom even though the old bladder was filled to capacity. I would get up all night long grunting and groaning just to see a small stream hit the basin. I became tied to the toilet. Well, like all good contributors to the medical institution, I went to a well-recommended doctor. He took X-rays and determined that what I told him to be true. Then he told me I had a few choices – surgery, surgery, and surgery. I found out about a process where they used a catheter burned on a larger hole in the tub and relieving the pressure from the prostate infection. I was told it would only last maybe a couple of years. Well, having had enough surgery with a steel-knee implant, broken neck, collarbone, etc., I opted for the temp solution as I talked to another person that had the same operation and was happy with the results. It's been six years as I have found a natural way of solving my problem.

I keep my prostate in top condition with my eating habits, parasites killing, and the application of my Beck Zapper. What's that? Hang on, we are coming to that wonderful invention, and it's great service to the health of all mankind. I was a victim, or shall I say uninformed sucker, for an unnecessary operation as I was the typical, naive American – product of the well-orchestrated media hype who thinks that all doctors are gods, infallible and have all the answers to all our health problems. I didn't realize like most Americans that a natural health industry existed and has been curing diseased prostrates for years without surgery. *"Natural Therapies for Prostate Problems" and prostate-miracle.com cover it all.* You just have to read all the materials you can on this subject before you subject your sex life and your reproduction glands to being victimized by the medical magistrates. My god, 180,000 people develop prostate problems each year, and major hunk of that group fall victims to the cut-and-slash philosophy that predominates the tactics used today with the medical elite. I could count on being a repeat victim at some later date. Well, that is all that it took to wake me up out of my slumber and complacency, thinking that if they can take my money, I'm going to get the best bang for my buck. Was I in for a rude awakening? I started reading and studying on what is really going on with my prostate problems. Causes and cures were not a part of the information I was given, and I was just curious enough to check it out on the computer. My fellow readers, the lessons of trial and error are a tough path to take when dealing with your own body functions. It was time for this old inquisitive man to take another approach.

Because of that little encounter with the medical cartel, I can safely say with some false pride, I have exhaustively studied and found alternate methods to keep the rest of my life off the sucker list of victims of medical ignorance. Parasites are the root cause of most prostate problems, and just burning a larger hole in the tube is not a solution or a cure. Kill off the invaders with the methods revealed in this chapter and you can easily retrieve prostate health.

One of the most important issues I want to program in your mind is the importance of setting up a maintenance program that keeps the parasites under control and incapable of destroying any of your organs vital for your survival. You cannot allow them to take up residence and control of your body. Read Web sites parasitecleanse.com, gifam.org, innerlifewellness.com, and curezone.com. Get well informed as you cannot know enough about these little critters that inhabit your body. We are on a parasite-control program and a personal-maintenance program that will change your life forever.

We will establish an environment in our bodies that is not friendly to all those little micro varmints that plague and threaten our existence on God's planet. Remember, they are survivalists and have existed since the beginning of time. So let's take control.

First line of defense is pure water. The body, being more than 80 percent water, needs constant source of pure water. The consumption of eight to ten glasses, eight to ten ounce, will greatly help in the reliving of ulcers, asthma, joint swelling, lower cholesterol; stop heart attacks; reduce pain, stomach disorders, high blood pressure – and this is only a partial list of the curative abilities of water.

Water also keeps the system flushed out and supports and prevents the buildup of toxic waste materials. Read Dr. Fereydoon Batmanghelidj's book *Your Body's Many Cries for Water*. We need to establish and maintain a regular program of flushing out our body systems as to be assured we're not drowning in parasites. There are many types of water combinations that are being developed like structured water, ozonated water, colloidal silver water, ADZ water, alkalizing salt water, and AT7 (fertilized water for plants). I use a combination of pure water, ozonated (ten minutes), ten drops of parasite killer, Dr. Clark's blend, and a dab of colloidal silver. I'm cooking this drink now before I go to bed. Have a ball looking up educate-yourself.org for some real excitement as to the new findings on the importance of using water as a natural stringent for the body. Just look at the small and down-to-the-point Web page of watercure2.com. Water intake per day should be one-half your body weight in ounce of water daily. I have 185 loveable pounds, so I try to drink three quarts of pure water a day with one-fourth teaspoon of Celtic Sea Salt. Keep a head close.

Now, the truth on parasite control with a simple natural application of silver colloidal water. I remember as a boy my grandmother making the statement about the few rich in our town of Austin, Texas, who had been born with a silver spoon in their mouth. She would put a silver spoon in our raw milk to preserve its time in our icebox as we milked our own cows in those days. Well, there have been documented proof that microscopic (nanometer size) silver particles suspended in water will kill upon contact over six hundred known species of parasites. This method of controlling disease has been used for hundreds of years.

Funny you have never heard of it, right? Taking homemade silver water will set up a natural second immune system to keep your body running at a top speed. This is a must to examine for your program of killing the invaders of our life force. Set up a maintenance program of making your own batch of colloidal silver, and take it at night before bedtime. I'm taking mine now as I am about ready to call it a day. Also, remember to drop in a few drops of black walnut and wormwood concentrate every once in a while, just to keep the buggers jumping and on the move. Fast and more ridged program is needed for the terminal ill, and you need to get a Dr. Hulda Clark book for that information. She has had hundreds of patients who have been cured of parasite infections. My program is geared to maintenance only as I have a seventy-eight-year-old body that has been abused by me for years. I now enjoy optimum health and a young wife who speaks for herself, so just keep tuned in.

When natural products are being marketed on the Internet, we always read a disclaimer that they have not been evaluated by the FDA. This means that no claims can be made as to the curative powers that herbs may perfect on humans before governments even existed. Herbs have to stand on their own merits without government approval. Herbs have been used longer than when the government existed, and somebody in the government needs to recognize their curative values and powers in sustaining life on God's planet. It amazes me how screwed up our representative system of government has become. I can remember when it was a government of, by, and for the people. Well, that doesn't exist today, and we all need to look after ourselves because government is on the take.

The present threat to the overall health of the human race is initiated from the greedy corporate elites who are fully aware of the need to curb population growth. The method they are using is selective as well as the targeted sectors of our populations. The affluent, educated middle class is their main threat to exposing their one-world agenda. This group is filled with naive Christian believers that God has prospered and protected. These people want to save the world and its people from self-destruction. They leave the management of the world in God's hands and hold no concern for the globalists' agenda of culling the world's populations into a manageable herd of one-third its present population. The greatest threat to mankind is their control of the medical and pharmaceutical industry. The globalists are making billions off your ignorance, their drugs, and your inability to cope with their new diseases of today. I am motivated to inform you, few readers who might enjoy optimum health in a polluted world. Nothing happens by chance, and contamination of our planet is taking place with your support and approval. The issues are ignorance and the avoidance of your government to confront these issues.

Most are aware of the growing problems in the world from overpopulation, food shortages, biological warfare, and criminals in Congress. Something has to be done; and since we the people are asleep, then the solution is being addressed by the antagonists, the globalists' elite money printers. This little book addresses the main issues and supports those of you who care to survive the coming world's manmade famines, plagues, and wars designed to bring the world under the control of a one-world globalist regime.

Being able to sustain your health from adverse attacks from biological warfare is one of our main goals in this book. That battle has already begun, just ask those living and dying in Afghanistan and Iraq. We have made enough dirty bombs (DU) in this world to kill the populations of the world ten times over. Bombs weren't made just to be looked at and stored in some underground safe place. Bombs are made to be used. Just ask the makers of the bombs. They will be used, and we have a group of world managers who have gone insane with their lust of power and desires for world control. Common sense is down the drain. Greed and power have taken control of these certain groups of mega rich, godless heathens who now worship power of the almighty dollar that they control. We are an addicted society and trapped with our temporal possessions. Our Creator is being mocked at churches as he has been reduced to an hour of attention on Sunday mornings. His words are being ignored. "You will reap what you sow." He has no voice in our media, our only form of entertainment, that is focused on violence and sex. News is a picture of our society gone amuck with killing, rapping, and disaster after disaster being the mind programming of the globalists to our populations. When was it last recorded that life on this planet was a godly experience with people learning to live peacefully while expressing love and respect for each other? All mankind should be working together for the general welfare of all humanity on the planet. Why can't we send food and cures instead of bombs and misery? I remember clearly when we were the most loved people on the face of this earth. How sweet it was traveling all over this planet making movies.

Americans were revered and loved. Yes, there was some envy; but I lived on their same level, and I easily made friends. We could go anywhere on this planet without the fear of being ridiculed or killed. I never see that world again. World peace will not return in my lifetime. The globalists' managers have pushed the world past the point of no return. There has been too much killing and destruction of so many nations. We have our corporate protectors (armies) in hundred and twenty countries out of the hundred and sixty that exist. We presently police most of the world while corporate America rapes all it resources. Would you like to change places with those Arabs living on that vast oil reserves? With our present mind of complacency because we can do nothing about the world situation, man just might become extinct. Don't think for one minute God takes kindly to that picture. He just might intervene and turn the table of events just to let you know he answers the prayers of Arabs as well as yours. This is not a political essay or discourse on world events, but this world does not belong to any self-ordained group of individuals who think they can play God because they control the wealth and resources of this world. It is just this one person's observations as I would like to survive the next ten years and watch the events that are being unfolded in our shrinking world today. I am not blind, and I do accept truth when I see it. The intimate goal of our world's elite is to enslave all humanity under fear and military control. That has never been clearer than it is today, even though most of the nations and their leadership are blinded and follow the leadership of the globalists who control the almighty dollar.

The globalists' money power has bought the loyalties of every country we now control and occupy, witnessed by our troops settled within their borders and the management of the natural resources a.k.a *oil*. Would you as Americans put up with ten thousand Chinese troops living down the street, looking after the Chinese interests in your once-sovereign nation? What do you think the last bunch of wars have been all about? The new so-called democratic nations are nothing but the pawns for the globalists. Their votes are a mockery to intelligence, just like it exists in good old America, the beautiful. You pay the large salaries of the political administrators who have added perks from their globalists so that their political futures are protected and secured. That's how the elite families control the affairs of mankind and corporate world.

What does this have to do with the health issue? Everything as corporate medical is all part of the world program for population control. Am I crazy? Lost all my marbles? If you control the medical applications of a society, you control who lives and who dies. Cancer treatments carry deadly side effects. Cancer patients can go into remission, but chemotherapy kills everything, the good and the bad – it doesn't discriminate. Are you listening to my plea for you to take control of your personal health? I pray so. *There is a parasite in cancer.* This statement was made by Alan Cantwell, MD, in his book *The Cancer Microbe.* The study of cancer being a parasite-infested disease was first discovered and proclaimed by renowned scientist William Russell in 1912. The discovery was named after Russell, and it is called Russell body.

Do you realize what this discovery means to the treatments of cancer? It appears that if you kill the parasite, you're able to put the cancer in remission. Isn't that exactly what chemotherapy does except it kills everything, good and bad, then destroys your immune system, and you're next to go? Cantwell called it a *cancer microbe,* and a number of data on this discovery can be studied in medical libraries. He proclaims "that there is no secret to cancer. The cause is right before our face in the form of Russell body. William Russell understood very well in the nineteenth century what medical science in the twenty-first century has yet to discovery."

If you have some symptoms of extreme pain and discomfort that seems to have no known origin, then your body is crying out for treatment. I am going to give you a list of some of the best books on developing good general health: *Peace, Love, and Healing* by Bernie Siegel; *Heal Your Mind Heal Your Body* by Joan Borysenko; *The Raw*

Energy Food Combining Diet by Leslie Kenton Food; *Your Miracle Medicine* by Jean Carper (food for cancer patients); and *Prescription for Nutritional Healing* by James and Phyllis Batch.

Now we need to summarize where we are at this time in our quest for obtaining optimum health. First, we must take control of our life and health. We are not guinea pigs for the medical profession. We are intelligent creations of God, capable of curing ourselves of any disease as long as we have access to valid and proven knowledge from relievable and creditable therapists and naturopaths. We have on the Internet all forms of knowledge to make a valid choice for ourselves.

Chapter 4

Detoxifying the Body

WELL, I DID it again. Just when I think I have my eating habits under control, I am up and fill the body with junk food and useless toxins. No ice cream though. This is my fourth trip through this book, and I keep adding and extracting data that I seem to have overstated to a point of boring even myself. This chapter is going to be the most important chapter in the book for one good reason. If we can keep the body relatively clean of toxins, allowing our body's natural functions will keep us alive and on the fast track. Remember, I try to have a mental hype to maintain the proper attitude; and in this chapter, it is very simple: "Whatever you can catch, you can get rid of it through detoxifying."

Fasting is the first simple, vital, and effective method of detoxifying the body especially when directed at long-term contaminants that have deposited their toxins in hard-to-reach regions of our bodies. Now is the time you may want to put this book down for a moment and browse through the following Web sites on fasting and detoxifying the body – hps-online.com and freedomyou.com. I used this method of fasting on water for cleansing my colon time after time; in fact, I just used it on that Thanksgiving garbage we had for our kids over the holiday – sweets, cola, candy, etc. Amazing how you can lead your kids to the water, but you can't push them in. No way I am going to convince them to eat properly. It would take an act of Congress and God to change their eating habits, and it's not going to happen.

I juice-fast for three days each month. It is one of the most effective methods of cleansing the intestinal tract I know. The reason is simple as we know exactly what we put into the system and, therefore, know what to expect. When I lived in Costa Rica, I routinely cleansed my intestinal tract as they played host to a multitude of health-destroying little parasites unknown to most Americans. Did you know that the hospitals in the States won't accept your blood as a donor if you have visited or lived in a foreign country in the past six months? Juice-fasting is relatively simple procedure as all it requires is a strong blender, fresh fruits, and fresh vegetables. Remember for the record, we eat to live, not to entertain our taste buds. Let the taste buds adjust to your eating habits, and your eating habits adjusted to sustaining your life on top of the earth.

Now this is my procedure for each morning of my life. This procedure is taken from well-documented data from various Web sites that I have posted. First and foremost, have your ozonated pure water with a heaping tablespoon of colloidal silver when you get up every morning. It takes about three minutes to ozonate a one-eighth-ounce glass of pure water. Also once a week, add five drops of 30 percent peroxide and ten drops of consecrated black walnut and wormwood product from NOW products at your local health food store. This gets the oxygen rolling through the veins and keeps the bugs at bay at the same time. Also, if you well along in your life cycle, you should be taking enzymes boosters as well as they help in the metabolism in your digestive system. These are recommended by Dr. Kelley at drkelley.com. You can get information from rainrocknutritionals.com.

They carry a fine line of products and less expensive than Dr. Kelley's line of products. It is important that they have that special enteric coating so that they are not digested in our stomach by strong acids but get into the intestinal tract to do the job of supporting the digestive system. That's your prebreakfast wakeup and the system water stimulator.

Now a half hour later, we get into our fruit-juice-breakfast-blended drink. We have total confidence and wonderful experience of using only fruits for breakfast up to twelve noon every day. We were taught this practice by Harvey and Marilyn Diamond in their book *Fit for Life*. Do not mix foods (water, carbohydrates, proteins, and fats) and don't put your system in stress mode in the morning with a lot of heavy mixed foods. So out went eggs, bacon, ham, pancakes, syrup, coffee, and the list goes on and on. We eat only fruits of all sorts in season until after twelve o'clock. Fruit normally requires one hour to digest except for bananas. That's why eating fruits in the morning is good healthy start to kick up the energy system for the day's journey. I believe it is well founded that as we get older and less active, we need less food to sustain our optimum life. Eating a humongous breakfasts in the morning just puts your body in the digestive stress mode most of the day, and the energy you would receive goes right back into digesting your food. Why should we waste vital quality time and money in overfeeding our bodies when we only need one or two meals a day to sustain our life with optimum health? Why not just take control of your eating habits now? Is it the herd instinct that pushes you to join the human herd of gross-out bodies at the feeding troth?

It makes no sense to stress out our digestive systems by overeating and forcing them to work overtime, trying to find nourishment in the junk foods you have consumed. Our bodies are just trying to keep us alive and kicking, reacting normally to the stuff we cram into our stomachs.

It just naturally starts hording and storing the excess fats and proteins you have eaten all over our bodies. I remember a friend of mine who had accumulated so much fat around his heart that he choked off his blood supply and died. You don't have to watch your weight if you're eating properly. Also, as we get older, we become less active and our metabolism slows down; so we are not burning up as much energy as we used too. What goes in must come out, and you need to monitor that process as it is your life on the line. Take complete control over all the eating functions in your life and watch carefully what you put in our gut.

Now I need to open up a real can of worms. The poisoning of our foods and bodies with heavy metals like mercury is the most toxic nonradioactive element known to man. You need to look into a well-informed and enlightened ladies the presentation of mercury poisoning of our populations (mercuryposioned.com). Please take the time to read carefully Marie's story and documentations on what the dental profession is doing to our populations with the practice of using amalgam fillings. Her Web page covers all aspects of dioxin and chelating the deadly poisons out of our bodies. Get rid of all amalgam fillings as soon as possible. Have them fill the holes with nontoxic substance that will not release deadly heavy toxins into your body. There are a multitude of excuses the dental cartel can come up to discredit this truth.

Mercury in your fillings is deadly, and you must get rid of it. There are a lot of other heavy metals that accumulate in our bodies, and we need to direct our efforts in the elimination of their terminal effect in our lives. We will now examine *oral* and *intervenes* chelating. Both of which are effective in cleansing the body of those stored heavy metals. (Vibrant Life Home Page covers all aspects of oral chelating.) Now, I am going to cop out on you as I believe if you determine your need to cleanse your body of heavy metals, then you need to read all the information you can digest before you make the choice on how to accomplish that feat. Purchase at the bookstore *All You Need to Know about Chelating* by Morton Walker. After you have read that information on this subject, you have sufficient knowledge to make a well-informed decision. If you're faced with a terminal possibility such as a heart dysfunction or the equivalent, then chelating is a must for your peace of mind. Remember, what Jesus Christ said, "Seek and you shall find, ask and it shall be given unto you." Don't overlook the need to detoxify your body of heavy metal contaminations. They can hide in your body and not really take their toil until we are older and our immune systems are overburdened. Once you have cheated the heavy metals out of the body, you relieve a large part of your immune system so it can focus on other essential functions and needs of the body.

Eat and live a well-regulated life by treating your body like it was the temple of the living God. A dwelling place for the living God who proclaims that "cleanliness is next to godliness." Purchase a variety of books for cleansing the body and do some in-depth research on the subject.

The more you know, the more you grow. Get more than one opinion on these important matters of cleansing the body as most natural food writers reach out for the same goals, but use different methodologies to obtain the same results. The more diverse knowledge you acquire, the more confident you become in the change you must make in your life. Be assured that the body is working on your side and will adjust to nutritious foods and helpful treatments in short order. Be ready to alter the program when the body rejects your first attempt. Every human is created in God's image. Just look at his creative qualities in the vast differences in the human races. Isn't that mind-boggling to see all the different races seeking and working to live in harmony with God and his creation? All accepting his or her own set of rules and customs needed for obtaining and living with optimum health. It sort of goes against my grain to see drug companies that program and test their drugs on one specific type of persons and then prescribe it for all humanity – young, old, black, and white. Is it any wonder that the drugs have to carry so many different warnings of side effects on so many different people? After all, it's doctors and drugs who kill most people in our world.

One of the best methods for detoxifying your body is eating natural, digestible, organic fruits with lots of water, allowing the natural elimination processes to carry and cleanse the body with all the accumulated hard-to-reach toxins. This could be a long-drawn-out process that you may not have the allotted time; but remember, the simpler the process becomes, the easier it is on the whole human body and side effects will certainly be kept to the minimum.

Choose the best and most comfortable convincing means to regain your health. This change of attitude may be really difficult to many people who totally rely on doctors as they have grown in a society where the media constantly pitches out, "See your doctor." Only the elderly can recall those days of living naturally with the bulk of their food being produced by local farmers. They did not have all the *dead food* of the fast-food industry or the *treat-all* massive drug industry. They weren't subject to all the massive health problems that we are confronted with today. How in the world could they exist without the local pizza parlor, hamburger joint, and chicken factory? Did you ever notice how these fast-food joints brag on how long they have been in the business of serving their toxic, synthetic foods to human life on this planet? None of them were here when I was kid. When you went out to eat, you got real home-cooked foods with a lot of natural nourishment and taste. The dinner out was a special treat of home-cooked food prepared by foreign chefs newly moved in from Europe.

Now the fruit juice I drink in the morning is one of the best natural colon and blood cleansers ever concocted – and the cheapest. All the fruits in season go into my drink along with frozen berries that I have grown during the season and kept in my freezer. The seeds contain a natural form of Laetrile (B-17), so don't take them out. Put a couple of drops of HCL (hydrochloric acid) to support your digestive acids and add a slice of lemon with the rind for a strong antioxidant. This fruit juice is very compatible to our digestive systems as it will digest in less than an hour while giving off welcome to early-morning energy.

When you eat fruits, your body isn't stressed out all morning trying to digest a lot of heavy proteins, fats, and carbohydrates all mixed together. You don't need coffee to keep the body stimulated and mind active. The fruit juice, along with the early-morning glass of ozonated pure water with silver colloidal water added every morning, starts the old body off with a good vital boost while giving the immune system and me a real sense of well-being. I don't take any vitamins in the morning as again I want the body restored on living off the natural foods it was created to consume. You might say I am reprogramming my body to live in its natural environment. Most vitamins I might need are found in the drink and the teaspoon of bee pollen. The rest I take in pills that I take along with my drink. You know, of course, that all humans worldwide enjoy eating fruits as part of their everyday staples. Men need fruits and veggies more than women as they require more energy to perform their functions in life as the breadwinner. Just look at the statistics: men have approximately one and one-half times the death rate of total cardiovascular diseases as women, one and one-half times the death rate of cancer, two times the death rate of lung cancer, one and one-half death rate of colorectal cancer, and two-thirds of men are overweight or obese. American has at least 58 million with some form of cardiovascular disease including high blood pressure. And 8.2 million Americans alive today have a history of cancer. Most of this can all be contributed to eating habits that have ignored the importance of eating fruits and vegetables as their main staple.

As you are probably aware by now, the cooking of food depletes vitamins and minerals and kills the essential enzymes needed for proper body metabolism.

Eating raw fruits and veggies will replenish that loss of those essential vitamins, minerals, and enzymes that my body needs on a daily basis. I could go into many reasons for this program, but one stands out above all the rest. The foods presently grown in America are devitalized because the soils have been depleted due to overuse and excessive leaching. Most growers today do not practice the age-old ritual of crop rotation as my grandfather did on our farm. They do not let the lands stand dormant for a year out of four. Even if the food is organic, it doesn't mean that it is vitamin enriched, capable of supporting optimum health.

In this chapter on detoxifying the body, we have many issues to address. We are greatly influenced by what we think of ourselves and our mental attitude toward our personal health. Self-imposed stress is due to the mind being focused on uncontrolled events in our lives that we have no control over. That stress rolls over into depleting our energy levels and causing abnormal pressure on all our vital organs in our bodies. We have stomachaches, headaches, body aches, and all kinds of signals that our systems are being overtaxed and depressed. Stress causes the adrenal glands to overload the body with alert signals that put the body on top of defense mode. Our nation of uninformed people have become complacent and satisfied with their health condition as long as they can function to some degree of efficiency. If it's working, don't mess with it is the attitude we assume toward our body functions. This mind-set should be addressed as we can't afford to fall prey to poor faulty habits, apathy, and complacency that overlooks pain indications as a frontal attacks on our body systems.

Do you realize that we are allowing our bodies to deteriorate because we are ignoring subtle signs and indications from the body that we are having problems with our life systems? The outcome is that we become depressed, reduced into a frightful subhuman existence before we finally wake up that we are wasting away. Neglecting your health is a mind-set, and if we continue to ignore the signals that the body puts out, it will eventually reduce our desire and energy to make the necessary change to save our lives. I call this a death wish, and I have seen it time after time with older folks. It's sort of like the obese person seeing himself as Mr. Universe. Our senses become dull, and we start to submit to living with an inferior life force that is operating well below the normal standard a life force should be lived. We might not even recognize this problem before; but suddenly, out of the dreamworld, we are awakened to the reality that are lives facing termination. This condition is brought about because of ignorance and apathy toward the needs of our bodies when the signals start to appear. We need to detoxify our minds as well as our bodies. Taking our health for granted and thinking we have nothing to concern ourselves over is like our nation sitting on a time bomb in this present polluted society. This is a must to read right now and even get a book (drrappmd@aol.com). The book is *Our Toxic World: A Wake Up Call,* and it will curl your eyebrows to read what has happened to our world and what is going on as disease is running rampant all around us and the hospitals are filled to the max. AIDS is out of control in many African countries and now in China. Virus, flu, and cancer are all around us; and we live in apathy and complacency.

Don't be discouraged if you find it difficult to be overly concerned over your health. It took you years of neglect that allowed your mind and body to be subjected to living in a subnormal physical state of life. It may take the rest of your lifetime to recoup your youthful existence, but you will witness improvements from day to day when you keep steadfast with your commitment. I have said over and over again, the choice is yours to make. How can I express to you how peaceful it is to go to bed at night with no pain, enjoying deep, restful sleep and an inner feeling of knowing that I am living my life to the best of my ability in harmony with all of God's creatures? I cannot express to you how comforting it is to know that my body is giving the respect it demands from my life with the choices I make. My body, mind, and spirit are in tune with universe; and we are experiencing a wonderful life full of rich and abundant joy that I have never experienced in the past forty-odd years of my life. I have started a whole new life cycle at seventy-eight. I call it "life after ignorance." I really enjoy sharing these newfound awareness to everyone's health support, even though I realize I have no qualifications or medical expertise to support the statements and findings that I articulate in this poorly written book. The definitions on health care tips I share are mostly my personal conclusions and are geared to the few who will listen to my babblings. I have had a broad personal experience in living this life and have been exposed to more life than I wish to reveal. Five or six of them before health enlightenment, living in the fast lane of Hollywood's mass insanity and under the corporate control freaks' manipulation of all media information.

I have never seen anything go into the pits of hell like the entertainment industry. The morals and basic values that was the core of our nation's success have been totally undermined; and all we get now is sex, illiterate numskulls, sick plots, violence, discrimination, and a constant demeaning of the Christian values of a Christian nation that gave us prosperity and prestige throughout the world. Women have been exploited and set up sex symbols for all to gaze and lust after. This debouched industry has developed all the sick new role models for our kids. Is it any wonder that our kids are so screwed up, going into our schools with guns to blow away our teachers? Is it any wonder we have more people in our prisons than all the other countries put together? Life in America today is rapid trip in an enclosed boat, riding down a raging river, headed for a thousand-foot drop onto a dry, rocky riverbed. My god, if that weren't so evident, I would not waste your time or mine with this feeble effort to persuade you to join me in this glorious pursuit for a healthy life. It is probably my last effort in this life to help a few readers in the restoration of health and plea for sanity to this nation of God-loving people. If we are to endure as a loving society, we will need to have souls who are not brainwashed and still remember our history when we the people lived with respect and dignity. We enjoyed having a government of, by, and for the people. Our government was designed to protect the values our forefathers established to secure our prosperity and freedoms. Our nation's Constitution was built to sustain our Republic and was not geared to combat traitors within our government. This new threat is all new to our people and needs addressing now.

We can't allow a handful of globalists to undermine and destroy our wills to remain free at all cost. We paid a price in the past, and we must be prepared to pay a similar price in the near future. This statement might sound a little trite, but I do have a deep vision and understanding as to what is presently happening to our once-free and open society. I visualize a lot of troubled times in the very near future as our present younger generation is being rendered helpless and brain-dead concerning protecting, guarding, and maintaining our freedoms. The new age teaching in our government-controlled school systems have totally voided exposure to our history and its founding fathers. The ideals and values that made our nation great have been omitted, and our heroes and role models of our past omitted from their books. The Constitution has become a myth and is no longer taught. As you can see, I am generally concerned of the future of our nation due to the fact we are becoming a nation of illiterates and blind followers who can be herded along like sheeplings. We are not exposing our young kids' minds to the Christian principles that our forefathers established for us to protect and sustain our freedoms. A new fascist, dictatorial society is being emerged and set up under disguise of the patriot act. The so-called middle class has all but disappeared, and the wealth of this world is controlled by 1 percent of our world's population. On my horse again. Back on my point, but I hope you can see that your health is a vital concern of mine for reasons beyond this simple explanation. Freedom is within, and it must survive with you as its guardian. Make it a point to get informed and prepare to stand your ground as the worst is ahead.

No person I know of has ignored, abused, and trashed their bodies more than I have. Apart from being run over by a stagecoach, having my neck broken by playing football, being dragged by a runaway horse, becoming alcoholic, taking drugs for years, and other enough debauched experiences to fill this entire book, I have lived a full, wonderful, eventful, otherwise notorious experience. I'm presently enjoying the healthiest experience of my life. Every new pain that comes up is a new challenge to eliminate naturally because it is only telling me that something needs fixing. It's like my old BMW when it creaks and howls, I know it needs looking after and I fix it as I can't afford a new one. I know it will serve me out if I look after it. If I can help one person to escape a miserable death at the hands of the practicing medical cartel and faulty drugs, who with good and bad intentions have totally ignored established natural cures, then this book is for naught. You see, the doctors are schooled in the state of the art of medical school factories that teach the methods of treating symptoms with drugs while totally ignoring natural causes and cures. The vision of a disease-free existence is not a fantasy or a figment of my imagination; it is a true, proven reality for thousands of souls who follow the laws of nature. Why do they, the medical cartel, not consider natural cures as well as that have been around for centuries? They are available to all and certainly are natural to the body. I mean, it is an added natural support to their drugs. The answer is very few, if any, are qualified to prescribe natural herbs to combat disease. They are not willing to put forth the maximum effort and time to get informed, and it would put them in competition with the pharmaceutical monopoly. Just a thought.

We are at war with big pharmaceuticals for our rights to have and maintain good health. In 1997, they spent 791 million dollars on television advertisement. This last year, they outdid themselves

COWBOYS UP | 191

by spending 3 billion dollars in advertisements, going direct to the consumers. Just read some of the facts on the battle that's pending for your right to have the information and access to safe and proven effective drugs. The FDA is under attack by us, the people.

Rep. Henry Waxman (D-CA) notes that the pharmaceutical industry is not keeping promises to conduct further safety studies of newly marketed drugs: a report delivered to Congress in March shows what happens with only 37 percent of regular drugs and 15 percent of biotech products pharmaceuticals are tested properly by formulation and quality (April/May 2002).

"It's shocking how can you say release drugs to the market sooner and not know it's killing people. It really is a dramatic statement of public priorities," said Dr. Brian L. Strom of University of Pennsylvania.

"Overall, the [pharmaceutical] industry alone has already spent more than $29 million in buying off politicians this year, more than any other industry," according to Political Moneyline, Fred J. Frommer, AP (October 14, 2003). "The committee and this Congress jump when the drug industry says jump: it rushes to pass legislation when the drug industry wants it to pass legislation. But we better not talk about the drug pricing or the impact of direct-to-consumer advertising on health care utilization. Those topics are taboo," said Rep. Sherrod Brown (D-OH) on March 6, 2002.

These guys seem to be good at getting their priorities screwed up.

"The United States is the only major nation that allows the private inventors of a drug or medicine to patent the discovery, even if it has been made with the help of a public grant and still retain exclusive rights to its production and sale thereby avoiding competition," declared Wayne O Leary (*The Progressive Populist*, August 1, 2002).

Looks like the drug industry operates without competition. Do you see why I don't support synthetic drug industry for curing our bodies.

It is the last resort for a man dying after he has tried all God's natural herbs. Sure they have some success with their drugs, but don't think for one moment they can replace God's natural products, compatible to our bodies. We should not take charge of our personal health, not the doctor that has ulterior motives. In summary, use a safe method for detoxifying your bodies of parasites by using natural products to do the killing and cleaning process. We can now live with complete assurance that each day we will get better, not worst. Life becomes a new experience as illness and death no longer have a stronghold on our lives. We are free from anxiety and stress that are major contributors to living with a miserable existence. I have been down that rocky road and know it well. I now have changed my focus on life and have included my Creator in all that, inspired to do with my remaining years. My simple prayer is that I will have the opportunity to help fulfill God's purpose for my sojourn on his planet. It is referred to as a divine calling on my life, and we all have one. Can you imagine after experiencing so much of life's best offerings, I still believe I have only touched the surface? Boy, there I go getting the cart before the horse as I will cover God's calling later on.

Chapter 5

Exercise Your Body and Spirit

Y OU KNOW WHAT they say about what you don't use? You lose. Well, this applies to the body as well as the spirit life in this case. Consider the fact that muscles are given to keep us mobile and able to perform work that supports our complex living styles. It requires muscles to do anything with our bodies. Looking after our physical bodies is obviously a major undertaking in the pursuit of optimum health. We are all aware that eating energizing foods will give us the mobility necessary to enjoy living on this planet. However, we have the antithesis to that if our flesh is not looked after with fresh blood to nourish the mire of cells. We will soon become invalids and subject to all kinds of body degenerations. Whose fault is that? We are in control of our body's physically activities, and it is our responsibility to keep the ship afloat. Modern comforts of life today are designed to make living in our advanced society soft and easy to all of us. We no longer have to plow the back forty, milk the cows, hoe the corn, or pick the cotton as I did as a child on the farm in Texas. We are a nation of complacent souls in pursuit of the enjoyment, looking for leisure time, watching television, traveling, reading books, and whatever entertainment we find to pass the time of the day. We are being cuddled from cradle to grave by our government-run agencies so that life has become an experience of complacency and apathy. We have given the big government full control over our lives. We are led to believe that we can't make a difference in government with our vote, but *we* the people no longer have any say in our government.

In fact, we have very little to contribute to the welfare of our nation, except sending our boys off to fight their wars of aggression. We are members of that vast herd called Americans that is being pacified and rendered brain-dead by media-proper gander into a planned, meaningless existence. We have compromised that godly quality within that needs to feel that his life has meaning and purpose to it. Without that assurance, he's a homeless vagabond that is blown to and fro with every storm, living without divine purpose for his life. Mankind has to communicate with his God for knowledge and the fulfillment of his divine purpose for in his life. Only his God offers that revelation as only the spirit of God can reveal it to him. The divine nature of God is to grant his creation the knowledge of his purpose in life. Animals have no problem with that godly instinct, only mankind. Something has to happen inside of man who turns him into a worshiping, humble servant of his Creator God. God sees his heart as well as the image implanted in his mind. There lies the solution to all man's inner anxieties as the world's religions reflect this basic need for mankind to find peace within that is an outgrowth of his belief system. It is reflected in all religions that the supreme creator has the key to eternal life. The godless heathens who set themselves up as like the Most High have to live with fear and anxiety over the outcome of their pending death. Fear controls their lives; they use that same method of fear to control the affairs of man. They can only control the unbeliever or godless heathen. Our planet's governmental systems have been taken over by organized satanic men who are possessed with fear of death and hell.

These elites live a subhuman existence as they can no longer enjoy their lives on earth. They are possessed by their possessions – fear from the power given them and discontented with the shallowness of their aimless lives. Their lives are entrapped with personal guilt and fear beyond explanation as they band together for comfort, mutual interests – solidifying their world aspirations. Fear like you have never experienced rules their lives, and they have no trust in anyone even the mass of servants they require to prefect their ambitions of world order. I express this fact not to enlighten you as to the problems the world faces, but for you to be aware of the power of fear and what it can do to your life. Anyone without an awareness of God's unconditional love in their lives live in constant fear of death and the unknown. Who am I and where do I belong and what is my purpose for existing always hang over as fatalism is their last resort. Nothing on this earthly plane of life can answer that for you, only your inner belief system that's wrapped up with your heart and soul can put your life, mind, and spirit at rest.

The exercise of our minds and our bodies are being opted out from considering our destiny by the carefully planned media machine that wants to entertain you from dawn to dusk and cradle to grave. Thinking souls are a threat to their plans for globalists' control. Meaningless entertainments of all kinds is the answer to keeping the minds occupied and focused on superfluous, meaningless trash that entertains the mind and pacifies the spirit. Like our behinds all day – hard labor, long hours, pushing keys, sitting at a desk, driving a truck, anything to meet the bills, and put bread on the table.

Some contend that we are living longer because we are not having to perform hard labor under hazardous conditions. We leave that most menial labor up to our illegal aliens. It could be true that mankind is living longer due to technology. However, are we living any healthier?

Somebody's illnesses are supporting a multitrillion-dollar medical industry, insurance companies, pharmaceutical industry, and a mire of doctors – but it's certainly not me. I haven't seen a doctor since I had my mercury amalgams taken out of my teeth.

Now enough of my rambling. Let's look at having a life free from disease and a good look at your heart. It's a vital part of your body that only operates for so many years without proper attention before it gets tired of being ignored and quits. You may not see the need for tuning up your muscles, but you certainly do have a need to keep the heart stimulated and pumping life-giving oxygen to all vital parts of your body. I haven't found a way to exercise the heart without putting muscles to work at the same time. So you just might have to learn to live with a body that has good muscle tone and works properly just to keep that heart of yours in shape. Heart disease kills one person every thirty-four seconds in the United States. You now understand that without a healthy heart, there is no way you're going to have an enjoyable life. I am asking you not only to eat the right foods but to do some creative exercising of some form every day. You need to have a set of plan to exercise your body. I go into contortions sitting in front of my computer in my swivel chair. I have invented some new movements that challenge this seventy-eight-year-old body. If it works for me, it can work for you. Just get the old body moving ten to fifteen minutes a day.

Your heart has to pump vital energy and oxygen to all parts of your body so that the trillions of cells can get the nourishment they need to function properly. Having said this, it is time for me to get on my treadmill to get my old heart moving again for I have been on this computer all afternoon and night. I'll be back in the morning, so don't go away. You know they say about teachers, you must practice what you preach. One more thought before I go. My workout takes about thirty minutes and another thirty in the sauna. I lose about five pounds of toxin-infested fluids. Did you know that foul body odor is a sign of excess yucky toxins in the body? Gross! Back again – all refreshed, little tired, and a few pounds lighter. By this time, you should have better understanding of what I call the commonsense approach toward optimum health. My parents both died of cancer with a lot of pain, suffering, and unpaid medical bills. It didn't take much persuasion for me to decide in my later years to take advantage of all the health-related information that is available over the free highway of cyberspace and books. What I really decided after seeing how my mother suffered as she did is that I would do anything necessary to live a healthy, pain-free life. And being a vain actor helped. So I am sharing information I have uncovered on this "beast" with all of you who would appreciate the fruits of my labors. Some time I am repetitive in my expressions, but that's old age, and I'm not so sure you hear me. I do have goals and a plan on how to accomplish and develop that commitment to my readers.

When I started this chapter, I wanted to demonstrate the bond we should have with our bodies and that godly spirit that dwells within.

We are body, soul, and spirit; and our minds have to be in tune with all the three for us to enjoy optimum health. This requires a spiritual awareness in our lives as we realize as created beings living in harmony with all creation that we must have respect and reverence toward all of God's life. Some one, some thing, and some force had a great imagination to create this world and all its living inhabitants. If you are a nonbeliever in a creator, that is your choice; but if you can conceive that a force greater than ourselves has established and maintains this universe and its millions of functions in perfect harmony, then we agree. I do not believe we have accidents in creation or big bang catastrophes. The universe has divine meaning, and there is a Creator God who is omnipotent, omniscience, and omnipresent and who regulates all factors of life to keep creation flourishing on the planets.

The most unique characteristic of mankind is that he can contemplate and give description to that force of creation. We can call it whatever we want, for labeling won't change it or its impact on the world. We are his created beings who have been given free choice, and we become the products of those choices we make. What we convince our minds and souls to believe and accept as gospel influences our life patterns, our thoughts, and the values we put to our belief systems. Who is to say that we are wrong or right? Our laws in this land are based on free choice and godly principles that were established by the God of the Bible. These same laws have made our nation prosperous and loved by all. Something powerful is transpiring, and my feeling is that our nation is leaving the Creator out of our lives and now worshiping the creation.

We idolize and covet all our temporal material goodies while ignoring their eternal source. Mental instability and stress have contributed immensely to most of man's diseases; however, I am convinced that without having a spiritual connection with your Creator is also detrimental to your health. Your Creator is the force behind creation, so he must be the force to restore his creation, including your health.

What I have chosen to believe has been influenced by my parents and many generations before them. I evaluated my belief system by the impact it made on my life and the health is has given me in that process. The values we accept for our lives and practice daily are reflected in all areas of our life. I am labeled a Christian by others as I am a follower of the teachings of Christ, which I struggle daily to apply to my life. I am not "religious" as I live with the belief that every person is a creation of God, and religions are notorious for separating and dividing us. Religion has been man's demise as more death and destruction has been caused by mankind trying to propagate his belief system at the threat of death and terror. Man's organizations are the means he can use to divide himself into like-minded herds that are compatible and driven by his desire to prove his philosophy is superior. Why does mankind always have a need to be approved or validated by his fellow peers for his spiritual beliefs as well as his philosophy of life? Shouldn't an inner confirmation and evidence of a lasting internal peace be enough to satisfy his spiritual and mental needs? Evidence of the need for peaceful existence is in the everyday, normal struggle in life. I have that with my wife as we have found peace and tranquility with praying together and being in tune with God.

Let me take that thought up a notch up and say evidence of being on the godly path with your life is apparent in your success at maintaining a peaceful coexistence with all God's creations around you. Instead of being created in the image of God, isn't mankind trying to create a God in his own image? Man's secular separation from a spiritual awareness of God is creating a factor in our society that is destroying any expression of God in our schools, governments, public places, and the world as a whole. Transformation will not come without troublesome consequences. Ignoring godly responsibilities that we as believers have been ordained to perform from our Creator will develop an inner anxiety and depression that will destroy our mental stability, homes, and families and reduce our lives into wandering herds of lost sheep. Take a good look at the society today, 38 percent of all marriages today end in divorce. I am a product of a broken marriage and barely knew my father who was a professor at North Carolina State University. My grandparents were given the burden of raising me and my brother as the Great Depression was still affecting our nation. I suffered from ADHD, which very few people knew anything about. I was a problem child who ran away from home and school, and the military institute was my parents' last resort to curb my problems. What they didn't realize is it was love and understanding that I was missing. That experience has disrupted my life and marriages that has caused me a lot of mental pain and insecurity. I have experienced eight marriages with kids spread all over the world. I am trying to catch up and get in contact with all of them now.

Carolyn is a big help, and we have contacted my brother Tex in Australia along with my son from my marriage to Lyndell who worked at the Playboy Club in London. She was a great gal, and I loved her to the best of my ability. When you take God out of your awareness, God will be forced to give you up to self-destruction. My marriages were a product of my ADHD, and the kids I had are victims of that disorder. You will have to get my autobiography book to get all that information as Carolyn is putting that together, and it will be coming out soon.

Now, after that "sermon," how does this relate to health? When the soul-spirit has settled this natural desire and need to find inner peace with his Creator, then spiritual and physical healing will soon follow. I am referring to the healing that reflects a peace that passes all man's understanding. Many refer to it as an inner glow or mind at peace with itself. I consider it as a stream of inner light that aluminates all God's creations, making this life experience a wonderful trip through time and space.

Last thought on this point is that we cannot separate the body from its soul-spirit. We cannot ignore the fact that there is a mind-body connection. One cannot do without the other, or our life will be filled up with chaos and susceptible to all types of negative attacks. Just as we are what we eat, we are also what we think. We must maintain harmony within and without. Seek a vision of higher awareness in your life and apply it to all that you do. My practice is to try to be aware of God's presence in my life and recognize his creative hand in all beauty that's around me. It's not always a pretty sight, but focus only on God's beauty. Read *Quantum Healing* by Deepak Chopra.

Chapter 6

Herbs that Heal

THIS IS A chapter that could easily take volumes to write. The study of medicinal herbs growing on this planet as food for humans could not be touched in this book as the study is massive. There are so many hundreds of herbs that are beneficial to our health. We are classified as herbivores; and our intestinal tract, being twenty-seven-plus feet long, is evidence that we are not meant to be carnivorous animals (herbmed.com). It takes four hours to absorb the nourishment from the digesting of herbs. Herbs are classified as natural plant life or botanicals, and that's what nurtures most life on this planet. Plants absorb carbon dioxide and give off oxygen that sustains all animal life on this planet. You might ask at this moment why I would bring up such a universally known topic. Life really is simple, and good health can also be simple, but we must be reminded that we make ourselves the victims of neglect and ignorance if we ignore the natural culinary laws of God. We have complicated our survival as we have ignored the basic principles of eating to live, not for the entertainment to our taste buds.

First, let's first address our principal problem of parasites. What is a parasite? It is any live organism that survives off your body's fluids in one form or another. There is a record of over six hundred various species that live within our bodies. Some are very helpful, and we call them friendly. However, there is a growing number of parasites (bacteria, viruses, fungus, and molds) that are deadly and have evolved to become immune to antibiotics.

Many of the parasites are so deadly that they can kill a man within hours if his immune system is vulnerable. Some are even flesh eaters, so we must take this message real serious.

Read "Germ Warfare Against America: The Desert Storm Cover-Up." This is not meant to be a scare tactic to propagate doom and gloom, but to send up a warning flag that emphasizes the seriousness of this topic. Have you noticed how much time TV news media is giving to deadly bacterial attacks? All types of new bugs out there are getting front-page news all over the world. Is that part of the terror that is being developed by sensational news reporting, or is it a fact? Parasites are a reality and will win the battle for our life if our defense systems become totally drained and ineffective.

We are being told that we might need mass vaccination of our population for smallpox, anthrax, etc. Government has purchased truckloads of these new vaccines from the drug companies and is now requiring the military to take them. What about the twenty or thirty other new alien bugs being exposed out there? Why secure yourself against one while you are being wiped out by another that has no cure and no vaccine. We have no time to build our immune system against it. Yes, that's what a vaccine does; it excites and prepares your immune system so it is ready for an bug attack. How wonderful our bodies are and how adaptable they can become with our help. But we can also ask ourselves how safe are the vaccines and what negative affect might they have on our bodies? Let's look at the difference between drugs and herbs. First, drugs are user dependent in that they don't cure but relieve symptoms.

Herbs, on the other hand, feed, build, and support our immune systems. Some herbs have the ability to kill the unfriendly bacteria that are feeding off our juices and life force. This is a complicated process as each herb has certain qualities that work on some conditions and don't work on others. Herbal knowledge is an art and a life dedication in itself. People all over the world have found treatment for disease from herbs in their own environment and have used them for centuries. "The herbs of the field shall be thy meat" (Gen. 1:29).

We are no longer living in our original habitats, so we have to look all over the world for medicinal herbal cures. I might add that herbs found in China might work on the Chinese, but may have little or no effect on us because of the differences in our body chemistries, blood type, and environmental issues. Some new herbs out of South America have done wonders for people in many cases. The drug cartel then finds a way to synthesize them and gets a patent so they can put them on the drugstore shelf. Why not maintain them in their original form rather than synthetic? Simple, because they just might be a cure for the illnesses and put their drugs out of business. Not good business from the drug company's point of view as it can't be patented and synthesized into a drug that has a hundred-year self-life. It is resourceful to create a product that the druggy can patent and market as a cure all for most anything you get and be sure and take it daily for the rest of his life. I know poker buddies of mine who have been on ten or twelve different prescription drugs daily, and they look like death warmed over. Some are drugs to counteract the side effects of others.

Let's talk about some of the herbs that are beneficial to support our immune systems. This is my daily program of supplements that support life:

1. Being seventy-eight now and reading all the stats on aging men having prostate problems, I take a couple of good prostate herb supports. I take my herbs and vitamins in the morning with fruit and breakfast. The product I used is Mother's prostate support soft gels with phytosterols. They use no fillers and are a good and natural product. I don't take vitamins at night as some are stimulating and may interfere with my digestive system, preventing a good night sleep. The herbs I take for prostate health are a combination of saw palmetto, uvaursi, bee pollen, buchu leaves, and zinc. Ginseng is a good replacement for male hormones, which are depleted as we age.

2. We've talked about colon cleansing previously, and the following herbs are at the top on my list for maintaining colon health. Look for these herbs in the cleansing formulas that you purchase at your health food store: psyllium seed, fennel, senna, peppermint, rose hips, cascara sagrada, oregano, rhubarb, and grape seed extract. Celery, watermelon, and bartlett pears are natural colon cleansers. Taking acidophilus, plane yogurt, or a good probiotic formula is essential to restoring the good bacteria in the intestinal tract after your colon cleanses. These are all natural ingredients that will assist you in keeping your bowels clean and functioning properly.

   Enemas should be taken in the morning just after your first bowel movement. I use two cups of organic warm coffee diluted with two cups of pure water mixed with two tablespoons of Epsom salts.

   I generally add ten drops of black walnut, wormwood, a combination of parasite cleans by Hulda Clark found at your health food store. Depending upon your self-analysis if you feel your body is in serious stress condition. Then ozonenate the mixture ten minutes and add two tablespoons of Epsom salts and insert into the colon for parasite extraction. I hold this concoction in my colon as I lay on my side for fifteen minutes or as long as I can. I change sides periodically and massage my lower abdomen with my hands or use a vibrator to help loosen the waste matter and encourage the fluids to move up my colon as far as it's possible. (I'm sure you all are excited about receiving this descriptive but vital information.) After taking an enema, it is a good idea to eat easily digested foods that support your cleansing action. After it's all over, take acidophilus, big swig, to restore the intestinal flora. Enemas should only be taken once every couple of weeks so as not to interfere with the normal peristaltic action of the bowels.

3. One of the most effective herbs to control parasites is an extract made from black walnut hulls, along with wormwood and cloves in equal amounts. This combination is a great cleanser for the intestinal tract and the entire body. I take this regularly, once a month for three days. I call that my body maintenance as it keeps intruders at bay. Suggested reading, *The Cure for All Diseases* by Dr. Hulda Clark, as it was her investigation that exposed this vital information. She is my hero and a real trooper.

4. I use lutein to strengthen my eyes as I'm abusing them constantly by my intensive use of the "beast" (computer). There are other herbs for the eyes like bilberry, eyebright, and grape seed extract.

    One of the most common causes of blindness in the elderly is macular degeneration, so a good eye support supplement is important along with exercises directed at the strengthening the muscles of the eyes.

    It is a good idea when reading to look up every time you turn the page and focus your eyes on something at a distance. The same method of exercise when on the computer. Staring at an object for a long period of time weakens the muscles and the focusing ability of the eyes.

5. One of the best, all-around herbs that has served mankind for centuries is echinacea combined with goldenseal for immune system support. You need to examine its usage and what it is able to do for you. It has been discredited by some, but it is well documented that it has a large scope of uses. Echinacea is one herb that should not be taken for more two weeks at a time. And goldenseal should not be taken by those who have an allergy to ragweed. All herbs because they are plants, have allergic potential, and should be discontinued if you develop a rash or any other allergic reaction.

6. Now for liver maintenance. Silymarin (milk thistle) and dandelion are two of the most common herbs use to support its functions. Look into a complete liver cleanse as it is essential for the elderly to maintain a healthy liver. At least twice a year, I do Dr. Hulda Clark's *Epsom salts* liver cleanse. This is a must for those who have lived in that fast lane of self-destruction. Look at the website health911. com as it has good products and very good all-around information. I like oil of oregano with olive oil for liver spots and warts that are fungus formations on our skin.

   Our livers cannot properly detoxify our intake of moldy old food and therefore deposits the mold on our skin. They can be removed but is not easy and takes time and patience. I'm working on that now with combination of the two oils, olive and oregano. So far, I am seeing good benefits, but it is still too soon to declare a natural cure.

7. There is a lot of talk about high cholesterol today, and several drugs called satins are advertised on television to "manage" the problem. What they don't tell you is that these drugs have been proven to diminish the body's supply of coenzyme Q10, which is essential for heart health. Dr. Julian Whitaker has brought this to attention in his newsletter and is trying to get the drug dealers to inform their patients of the necessity of taking coenzyme Q10 as well if they find it necessary to take the drugs. However, there are natural means

available to help to lower cholesterol without side effects. Eating plenty of fiber and taking *omega-3* essential fatty acids (EFA), lecithin, niacin, and garlic are all helpful in naturally reducing cholesterol. Something you need to look into if you seem to have a chronic cholesterol problem is a change in diet.

8. For a blood cleanser, burdock root is one of the best. One of the most informative Web pages on the Internet for herbs and their usages is herbalformulas.com. Look to set up a maintenance program that works just for you as all body metabolisms react differently to things we eat. Herbs carry enzymes that support various functions of our bodies, and we need to explore all those options in our pursuit for optimum health. What that could mean is that we could survive and treat all deficiencies on herbs and plants alone.

We only need to be schooled on which herbs are adapted to our bodies and offer us the nutrients needed to support our immune systems. Nature has the perfect formula to your body that you got to find it in all the natural products rhetoric and I will share mine with you; but unless you're a seventy-eight-year-old, six-foot-two-tall, and 185-pound English aristocrat and a Texan cowboy, it's useless to you. Somewhere out there in cyberspace, there are perfect herbs that support and grant you optimum health.

Another thought for this chapter on God's natural cures is the daily use of pancreatic enzymes that support the work of the pancreas which is essential to digesting food. Dr. Kelley's book, *Another Cure for Cancer,* that you can download on the "beast" will inform you how to keep the body functioning properly and maintain good digestive juices. This is vital information that has been kept from the populations of the world. Every person can use this information.

Let me caution you that herbs can also be toxic and harmful if not taken properly. Many herbs need to be taken only when certain conditions mandate, and not all the time. Some herbs interact in a negative way with prescription drugs, so you need an in-depth study on what ails you followed by the same approach to what will cure you. I am working on a cure and maintenance for cancer cells, and I have it right now. I will excerpt my maintenance program in the next chapter if I remember. I came across a very informative book I use quite frequently, *Prescription for Nutritional Healing* by James and Phyllis Balch. Lots of good people are trying to right the injustices the pill doctors are peddling to victims.

Chapter 7

Mind Over Matter

THIS IS SOMETHING off-the-wall, and I will briefly discuss what I refer to as mind control. So many of our fellow inhabitants on this planet have become what I refer to as TV brainwashed, medically duped, and victims of a clever media hype. They are unable to think objectively for themselves. We are a trusting, benevolent audience of freedom-loving, Christian-based people who are inclined to believe everything we read and hear by the overwhelming promotional techniques of our present, carefully controlled media. Everyone is selling something for profit. We have been programmed to accept what we are told without seeking another opinion or questioning the sources.

We have become a nation of pacified, complacent optimists who think everything is going to work out all right . . . just leave it to our elected representatives and everything will work out in the long run. I think they call those folks eternal optimists or brain-dead mummies. Well, that might be well and good within our family units, but that's not the real world we live in today. Everybody's on the make, and money is the motivator. It has become a world of the fittest survives and the almighty dollar directs the affections of mankind as a whole. Money power has become the object of man's affections, replacing our God who is now reduced to hours or so on Sunday morning.

Lets us be honest for a moment. What is the prime motivator of our present society? Seeking all the worldly possessions and creature comforts, we can obtain before we pass on. "He who dies with the most toys wins the game."

We have a society trapped in debt focused on sustaining his lifestyle and worldly treasures in fast-faltering society. While he has been obtaining the world's temporal goodies, he has become blind to the true values of life. He has lost sight to the values that made our lives and country meaningful, productive, and loved by most all the world. Is it any wonder now why our society is feared and envied by the rest of world? We are a sick society, building a massive arsenal of weapons to destroy the world's habitation. We are greedy and lustful in our desires to control humanity and cull masses of populations worldwide, and we will use any means we have to do it. We are out of control with our power over this planet and have lost our Creator God. Do you not think for one minute we won't *reap what we have sown*? This is not a healthy situation we are being forced to live in. We have become the scourge of the planet.

My dollars, like most Americans, have taken a real turn to the bottom of the stack after 9/11; but as I see it now, it may be a real blessing in disguise. I am more focused and determined to improve life conditions on this planet than pursue the almighty dollar. I have left the film industry, which is a mockery to our values and Christian nation. I now want to share all the experiences and lessons that I have struggled all my life to learn. Through these seventy-eight years of hell I put myself through, I have come out on top. That is a miracle of God as only he could live with my self-destruction and health assassination. I am now redeeming undeserved grace from my God so that others can possibly gain from all my blunders. The second most important issue of life is optimum health. God is first.

I have since childhood had a disease called ADHD. A long-term disorder that has brought on massive confusion and undue anxiety that has given me grief beyond belief. I have aimlessly wandered all over this planet for over seventy-eight years. It has been impossible for me to stay focused on any project long enough to complete or accomplish anything of value or meaning. The book I am currently writing with my present wife of a year (if it ever gets finished) will be an extensive study of my life and focuses on exposing my ADHD as well as all my wives and children that are scattered all over the world. It also reflects my career in Hollywood along with my marriages and children. I am the prime example of this disease run amuck as it has wreaked havoc in my life for sixty-five years.

The purpose for me bringing this up now is that I have been a part of that entertainment media blitz that has addicted its viewers, programmed their minds, and turned them into puppets of the globalist agenda. We all fantasize as we become involved with our favorite form of entertainment and enchanted with the stories that affect our lives and thinking. Many wives who stay at home live with the soaps while their husbands are totally involved with sports programs and the local bar. We are all accustomed to being entertained by a media that cares little or nothing about the wholesome Christian values we endorse in our society or did. The quality of the garbage we are absorbing is not fit for human consumption. Many of these programs have subplots that are being used to undermine the basic moral Christian values of our nation.

What would happen within our society if we stop just listening to others and become truth seekers and freethinkers? All societies must have a higher vision and purpose for life. Mankind must begin seeking higher awareness and peaceful coexistence with all creation. We are coinhabitants of this shrinking planet that is fast becoming polluted by greed and indifference to nature's laws. That mentality must stop now, or the repercussions will be devastating. We may have passed the point of no return. Instead of finding ways to annihilate our so-called adversaries, we need to find ways to live in harmony with each other on this planet and realize we are all brothers of the human herd. War begets war, and bombs are built to be used. Where does it stop? We are all to blame for 9/11 as it takes two to tango and two to make war. The effect is never separate from the cause. We know that there are differences with our Arab brothers, but they can be solved by sane people who put God's laws above their own.

We will probably be at war when this gets printed. But why aren't governments trying to find the means to work out our differences? Does history always have to repeat itself over and over again? We never seem to learn from our mistakes. Does man's unshakeable desire for power and greed always override his application of experience he should have gained from his mistakes he made in the past? Is his future history going to be a remake of his past? If so, we are doomed as we cannot afford another world war even if the elites do have their underground cities. What a total tragedy mankind has made for himself on this planet! Can anyone put some common horse sense into the globalists?

What's more important now is to reach the servants of these global idiots and have them stop the destruction of our planet. Stop committing massive injustices against the common folks of our society. Police and armies have to stop serving the interests of these globalists and killing off innocent men and women to protect their unjust laws that are geared to culling off millions of the world populations.

Think for a second what would mankind gain if he lost the whole world to nuclear fire and ashes. It is insanity to think that we can gain peace on this earth by threatening and intimidating whole populations.

Those who would continue this plan for world domination are in for a real awakening as it cannot and will not happen as God will intervene and evil men will be tossed, if they think they can take control of his planet. There exists a loving Creator. Look at what he created, and he surely will intervene against any injustices that threaten the existence of his planet and its primary resource – human life.

Social reformers must first eliminate their own ignorance and educate themselves on the basic causes of insanity and remedies for those social disorders. This includes the economics, politics, and ethics of the problems and their solutions. To remedy social ills, you must replace ignorance, apathy, and greed with knowledge, empathy, and charity. When the masses are aroused with empathy and armed with knowledge of the remedy, the few greedy opponents will either sway themselves to join the righteous battle or be overwhelmed by the greater force of the righteous revolution. You can see the need for freethinkers, not subjects, to proclaim the means and methods to bringing about world peace.

This is a time in history for mankind to restore to his natural state the art of seeking his Creator's purpose for this human experience. Most societies are doing this in one form or another, but rulers have become so focused on the creation that we are sidestepping the Creator. It is my belief that God's perfect plan never includes violence and wars that kills, maims, and destroys his creation. The soul of mankind is precious in his sight as he desires mankind to be with him in eternity. Why not, he doesn't do anything without a divine purpose, right? Where is it written or decreed that there are different values put on certain souls that grants them more importance in the sight of God and grants those souls the right to exist while others do not. "The meek shall inherit the earth" is in my Bible even though I've had no time seeing it. "Blessed are the peacemakers" – that one I can and do work with better.

Chapter 8

The Body Electric

YOU'RE GOING TO love this chapter. It is one of my favorites, for it utilizes some of my almost-forgotten skills in the field of electronics. After my education at Texas A&M University, I went on to work for Douglas Aircraft Company in Santa Monica, California, as an acoustical-electrical research engineer. The DC-8 needed a suppressor to knock down the noise levels that keep from tearing off the tail. So here we go, and I hope you will understand where I am coming from. This study is about the cleansing of our bodies from parasites with the use of electrical and magnetic potentials that is called zapping.

Our society kills and condemns humans in the electric chair with the use of megavolts of electricity. They literally fry the body to death by killing all the cells in the body. Our bodies require and retain salts, so we become very good conductors of electrical impulses that the brain sends out to all parts of our body. Those impulses are used to activate all body functions. One could say that our bodies are the most complex computers in existence. We inhabit a body that has the most advanced signaling system in the whole world. Our mind is constantly in communication with all parts of the body without our conscience's participation. The body is always in tune with the mind when something is not right and pain indicates a malfunction. Now, that same brain goes to work to trying to find a solution to solve the problems. The body's subconscious mind then sends out a host of support units to combat the intruders. The body has many options he can choose from in order to defend and destroy any foreign entity that desires to feed, destroy, or harm any functions that preserve and sustain our lives. Self-healing always precedes physical applications. If the body is short of resources, stressed out, and overloaded with toxins and disease to defend itself, it will cry out loud for your support. This preservation of your life is an ongoing battle, and our body's defense mechanisms spend very little time resting, that's why having a good sleep is imperative. Your body maintains vigilance over your organs and health twenty-four hours a day. It needs all the help you can give it. It is designed by God to maintain your health; however, it can use all the support you can give it, especially that as we get older, immune systems shot, and we neglected the laws of nature.

With this being said, what else can be done to support the work of our bodies? We have previously discussed the importance of proper eating, so now we need to do a little precision killing, which will rid our bodies of undesirable inhabitants known as parasites. These micro-organisms are the cause that most illnesses in our bodies release toxins that destroy our life force after feeding off our resources. The battle for life is an ongoing epic that becomes dramatic as we age; body weakens, and bugs get more aggressive.

In the fall of 1990, two medical researchers working at Albert Einstein College of Medicine in New York discovered that by applying a low-voltage, direct current electrical potential to blood by using two electrodes, viruses could be rendered ineffective and destructible by the body's immune system. This was a milestone in disease control and understanding. After the initial announcement in various newsprint (*Science News*, March 30, 1991, p. 207), Dr. Bob Beck saw the article and realized the immense value of this technology. He went on and developed it further as he realized its potential in curing disease. Every living organism gives off its own resonant frequencies. By laboratory testing those frequencies and having knowledge of the potential to counter that frequency, one could kill the bacteria by using plasma wave radiation. The bugs would literally, internally shatter and eviscerate, thus destroying it. By this means, he discovered that it is possible to rid the body of all parasites, fungus, and viruses by knowing and testing the resonant frequencies of the parasites. The process doesn't happen overnight, but it is possible to witness change in the body's energy levels right away.

I have watched my own hair slowly thicken as it's turning to all gray, and my energy level has increased twofold. I can testify strongly that it works for me and hundreds of others. There is much evidence on the value of magnets applied to the body for healing and the reduction of pain. I use a magnetic belt sometimes when I go to bed as I have a tendency for lower back pain. With the belt, it is always better in the morning. I would suggest that you educate yourself on a magnetic healing as we live in a magnetic field that surrounds our earth. It appears to enhance the quality of our blood by magnetizing it. I also use magnets attached to a funnel as I draw water for drinking. Lourdes in France has magnetized water that has proven to be beneficial and healing for mankind for hundreds of years. If you are interested in reading more about this, I would suggest a little book entitled *Magnet Therapy* by Ghanshyam Singh Birla and Colette Hemlin. Quantumbalancing.com covers it all.

Ozonated water is water by protazone that has an extra oxygen atom (O_3) attached to it, making the water very instable, thus releasing beneficial oxygen into the body. My day starts off with a glass of ozonated water with a little colloidal silver. Now let's also consider ozonated olive oil and its curative properties for killing bacteria that have settled into hard-to-reach areas of our body. I do not have enough room to put down the great amount of usages that this therapy offers your life. Look up cansema.com on the Net for skin cancer and other skin treatments. I use ozonated olive oil mixed with oregano oil to keep my ears free of fungus and to eliminate liver spots.

Hydrogen peroxide therapy has been developed by many fine doctors, one of whom is Dr. Kurt W. Donsbach who has documented the results of this type of therapy. When a disease lives without oxygen, it is said to be anaerobic, like cancer. These diseases will die in the presence of oxygen, so we can see how important it is for our bodies to have access to an abundance of oxygen. This paragraph may be short, but it carries a real wallop. It is a therapy that I use on an as-needed basis. It has been proven it will destroy the newly developed bugs. AIDS, released in Africa, was killing millions of the black populations. Oxidative therapy technology has proven successful against AIDS in all the cases recorded in a pamphlet entitled *Hydrogen Peroxide Therapy: New Hope for Incurable Diseases* by Conrad LeBeau.

Getting back to ozonated water, I would like to encourage you to purchase a water ozonator to use daily in your water consumption. I use my ozonated water to put oxygen directly into my blood system every morning. This extra oxygen goes directly into my brain to help with ADHD and assists me in good decisions for the rest of the day. It works wonders for me, and I feel its effects as I am writing my autobiography. I need my head clear to recall my life's history and write this booklet. So much water has gone under the bridge for this old man. Fortunately, my computer does my spelling for me, even when it can recognize the word. Without my lovely wife's assistance with her proofreading and support, this game plan was over before it got started. Folks, I know by now you think I'm some kind of quack, but the ozonenated water is a must for us oldies.

Chapter 9

Second Immune System

W E ARE GOING to talk about another technology that was developed thousands of years ago, but has been suppressed by our elites. In the past, we referred to the elite as being raised with a silver spoon in their mouth. This expression refers to the fact that they used silver utensils and also used silver to keep food from going bad, such as milk. They would drop a silver coin in a container of milk to preserve its shelf life. Silver is a well-known antibiotic and was used by our forefathers for centuries. As far back as 4000 BC, Persian history records using silver vessels to store water. The Romans reported using silver compounds for medical treatment. The March 1978 issue of *Science Digest* called silver our mightiest germ fighter. Dr. Harry Margraf stated that "silver kills some 650 different strains of disease organisms."

According to the encyclopedia, "the element silver exhibits bactericidal properties not fully understood, although these are thought to be a result of its inability to absorb oxygen. Colloidal silver is used as an antiseptic germicide, astringent, caustic, for water sterilization and to arrest hemorrhaging by coagulating the blood. Astringents act by shrinking tissues and reducing the permeability (passage of gas or liquid) of membranes. They may be used internally to diminish mucous secretion in a sore throat, check diarrhea, or reduce stomach acid secretion. Externally, they are used for conditions such as cold sores, poison ivy, hemorrhoids, and as an antiseptic eliminating rashes, odors, disease, and odor-causing microorganisms." This is found in thetruthseeker.com; I like this.

Colloidal silver preparations are used as antiseptics, particularly for application to the mucous membranes of the eye, nose, throat, urethra, bladder, and colon; and they are commonly used to treat infections of the upper respiratory tract. Twenty-three colloidal silver preparations contain a high concentration of silver, largely in the non-ionized form. Their antiseptic value depends on the activity of the free silver ions and not on their content. They do not precipitate protein but penetrate the tissues and are extremely toxic to all bacteria and parasites.

The drug cartel developed antibiotics that kill only six to eight types of bacteria (bugs). Colloidal silver is documented to destroy almost all bacteria along with the simple infections, viruses, fungi while protecting the natural enzymes of the body. It is a known fact that many bacteria are developing immunities to modern, specialized antibiotics at an alarming rate. The *Los Angeles Times* reported on October 23, 1994, that "bacteria can transfer genes among themselves and experts expect the resistance to grow." University of California, Los Angeles Medical Center has reported that colloidal silver killed all virus that was tested, none of which were immune.

Colloidal silver consists of molecules of pure silver suspended in pure drinking water. It is made by driving electric energy across two silver poles submerged in water. By setting up two poles of pure silver tied in a series in a glass of pure water with a simple eight-volt DC battery, you can produce your own colloidal silver. The product is sensitive to light and heat; therefore, storage of colloidal silver should be in a colored glass jar in a dark place. It takes twenty minutes to make a quart of colloidal silver light gold in color.

If you don't want to make your own as I do, this product is available over the counter in most heath food stores.

Now with regard to application, I will only relate my own personal use of the product. You need to look into the references and read some of the more important articles that I have included on the reference page. I take a large mouthful every morning I remember to do it. I hold it in my mouth and gargle with it for a minute as I have all my teeth still in place since I started performing this ritual. Then I put another ounce in my ozonated water to drink with my morning supplements. I also have two reusable nose spray bottles that I fill with colloidal silver and use them on my eyes, nose, ears and scalp when needed. The small silver particles penetrate the pores and eliminate whatever micro adversary that is causing irritation to my skin. There are more uses than you can imagine or that I can put in this little book. It's great in your enemas. By applying colloidal silver to my scalp. I am hoping for the best but am satisfied with not losing any more hair. This has also been documented by those other than myself. There is no more hair loss, and that alone is worth shouting about. I keep the nose spray bottles by my bed at night to use as needed to clear a stuffy nose. I have no more need to purchase over-the-counter drugstore nasal sprays, which are proven to have addictive qualities. Ask your pharmacist or go to theft-by-deception. com. Just plug this in for fun and be creative with you health.

Colloidal silver is a product I would strongly suggest taking the time to read all the information on it you can find. I call it my second immune system or my *antibio protection shield.*

The FDA has labeled colloidal silver a pre-1938 drug. That alone says a lot for its value and importance to your health. It may be become especially useful in these times with the threat of world bio-warfare and new microorganisms, deadly viruses being introduced into our society on a daily bases. This product, after you have set it up for yourself, may be God's answer to terrorism within and without.

"All truth goes through three stages. First it is ridiculed. Then it is violently opposed. Finally, it is accepted as self-evident" (Arthur Schopenhauer).

Chapter 10

Third Immune System

THIS IS A very small paragraph on *urine therapy*. It is not very popular subject and is not practiced by a lot of people because of the nature of the beast. It is not a common practice to drink one's own urine for health purposes; however, the evidence and material on this therapy is overwhelming and cannot be ignored. There are many Web pages on this topic that substantiate the benefits of this little known practice. For anyone with cancer tendencies, it's a must to look up. There are over 254,000 pages on this topic on the Internet and a lot of documentation to substantiate this therapy as a viable means of treatment. I might add that I haven't gotten that sick yet to give it a go, but you can bet that I would if I had no other choice.

Writing this book has been a highlight for me and has given me so much satisfaction and enjoyment knowing that I am able to express and give witness to the wonderful gift of good health that I am fortunate enough to live and experience. I have made it a priority to share with those around me the ideas to improve their quality of life and how it has worked. I'm praying that my firsthand observations might enable you to help yourself and others who would enjoy some form of physical comfort in their own lives. Try starting off with a change in the diet, ridding the body of deadly chemicals added into foods that preserve their shelf life indefinitely. Set up a proper schedule of taking the proper supplements needed to support your immune system. You never want to take over the body's functions, just support them with proper organic pills. I'm trying in some small way to alter the belief that only the allopathic doctor has the ability to treat disease when there are many alternative methods of treatment available to accomplish this feat. For the most part, the mainstream doctor has only been taught to treat the symptoms with drug therapy. The fact remains that the body heals itself as long as we support it and give it what it needs to perform that feat.

My objective here is to try to assist common folks in knowing for themselves what is good, sound therapy to assist the body's natural curing ability. To acknowledge that they have choices for the course of action they take for obtaining optimum health. The body is flexible and can adjust to our determination to do what is proper and beneficial for its health. Knowledge is the power over medical blunders, and healing always starts within the mind.

Millions die yearly at the hands of doctors for various excuses. Like administering the wrong blood type, wrong medication, wrong diagnosis, and the list goes on. Doctors are well protected with their liability insurance. Limiting the importance of the doctor out of the equation of self-healing and filling it with knowledge, intuition, common sense, along with godly instincts, you now got a winner.

Many doctors are having to close down or are putting a limit to the Medicare patients they treat. Malpractice insurance costs are so high that doctors are being forced to price themselves out of business. The doctors are calling for legislators to put a limit on the amount of bucks the victims can sue for. Now, who profits from this one? Will the doctors be a little more conscientious about their prescriptions and practices, or is this a move to protect the insurance companies from the families of the victims? Who supports the leeches in government, corporate America, right? I'll put my money on the insurance companies. My heart really goes out to the victims, the patients, who needed professional help for his diseased condition and got neither.

We need to understand what freedom truly is and what it is not. The freedom of choice can only apply when one has options available to him. When corporate greed takes away man's options, then his vote is worthless. Drug companies are now telling Canadian pharmacies they can no longer sell prescription drugs to Americans because they are cheaper in Canada. They are being threatened with the loss of product if they continue to sell to Americans. Who are the victims in this case? Many seniors, on fixed incomes and without prescription coverage, have been making the trip to Canada.

Why are prescriptions so much more costly in the United States? It's as though we as American citizens are being penalized by our drug corporations for wanting to stay alive. Something is drastically wrong with our system as so many folks cannot afford their drugs. If you're one of them victims, let me know, and I will send you this book for free. I am livid that our elders are being ripped off by greed from the pill pushers and nobody cares.

Why have the drug cartels become so powerful and so rich? Why have we become a nation of diseased and dependent souls addicted to the prescription industry with there mass media advertising propaganda? Do you have any idea how much it costs to underwrite a television show like Bronco by paying for the advertisement? Is there any wonder why we are charged an arm and a leg for drugs, doctors, and health care supplements? Greed and power are out of control in our world. The world is out of tune with reality and is on a path to self-destruction.

No one wins when the whole system collapses into total chaos and life no longer holds any value. No peace can be sustained in a society that lives in total financial bondage.

We must revive love and concern for one another and find compassion in our hearts for all mankind, especially our elderly. Not promote them out of their lifesavings. The elderly are naturally fearful of dying or suffering in their last years on earth. Why have the medical establishments target this group of citizens? The lowest form of human life is those people who now target helpless souls that are in need of valid treatments for cures after they have dedicated their whole life preserving this planet for his prosperity.

Whatever happened to that caring family doctor who sacrificed and traveled great distances at his own expense to alleviate the suffering and pain of humanity?

A change in the course and direction of our world is a must if we are going to sustain human life on this planet. I have no desire to live underground even if I were invited. We need to restore confidence and creditability into the medical profession by seeking to move the treatment of disease to natural homeopaths and informed citizens who practice natural restoration of the body. We must restore creditability and compassion in and for each other, which starts with you and me. Your health is of your own making, and cures are offered as long as you have access to valid, pertinent, and reliable information that can be affordable. So much of our elderly population is strapped with irreparable debt to the pill pushers. Health care is not affordable to the elderly, and their lifesavings are in jeopardy when they walk into that doctor's office. As long as there is a glimmer of freedom of the press in our nation, you can find men and women willing to subject them to ridicule and persecution just to preserve the right to offer valid information on self-healing. The Internet offers many proven established cures along with disinformation to create and develop confusion and doubt. You must seek God and ask for discernment to dissect the truth from all the misinformation that is available to the gullible.

You can enjoy relatively inexpensive health care by helping yourself to the free information on the Internet where I have found good, God-fearing men and women willing to share their knowledge for curing disease naturally.

Information published in this book was gathered in love and concern for my fellow men. I wish it were more conclusive and specific, but then the quacks would get all over me. We still are very fortunate to be living in a land of so many God-loving people who will go out on the limb to help his neighbor and restore our Constitution's government.

Millions of souls out there are seeking to understand as to what is going on with this world. Why is there so much misery and killing of God's creation? Why do so many people in this world despise and envy us, and why am I bringing up this controversial issue at this time? Because inner spiritual peace has a direct effect on our overall health. Health starts as a mind-set, and we begin recovery from illness by the healing of our mind-body experience in this life. We first must believe that we, as a nation under God, are going to be healed by doing everything we know we can do to support and preserve peace and harmony both within and without the world. That is positive thinking at its best. That is the vision I carry for my own personal peace and our constitutional system of government, knowing that good and honorable men will rise up in time of trouble, and God's established nation will be sustained. Paul Revere was born on January 1, 1735; and I was born on January 1, 1930, two hundred years later. Paul rode his horse to warn the people of the coming storm. I have retired my horse, but the message is the same. Folks, time is running out, and we need to find the means to restore our constitutional government. My plans are simple. Get informed, get armed with the power of God's Word, and get our pastors to read the Bible. We are facing the end-times.

Closing Remarks and Summary

NOW IS THE time to get to the bottom line of this effort to present information that can speed you on your way to achieving optimum health. The following is a list of books that I personally recommend for your reading. They have valuable information on the subjects we have discussed in the previous chapters. With an open mind, this information will establish and secure your life on the path toward your own personal health program.

1. *The Cure for all Diseases* by Dr. Hulda Clark, PHD, ND. The first of her books that shook medical establishments. Dr. Clark has endured a multitude of abuse from the establishment just to bring you the remarkable truths regarding herbal treatment and general health. A real saint for our time.

2. *Cure the Incurable* by Dr. William D. Kelley, DDS, MS. A book on the treatment of cancer. This book can be found on the Internet or in your health store. A great survivor of God's army of compassionate souls and a real defender of the truth. Defines cancer scientifically. Note: I take digestive enzymes every morning of my life as he

recommends. They must contain trypsin and chymotrypsin, or they're useless as far as this doctor is concerned.

3. *Prescription for Nutritional Healing* by James F. Balch, MD. This is a great handbook for self-help and your home library.

4. *Super Health* by Dr. Donsback. Another must for truth seekers and health freaks like me.

5. *8 Weeks to Optimum Health* by Andrew Weil. Just makes good sense with deeper knowledge to obtain. The more you read, the better you can discern truth by yourself.

6. *Bypassing Bypass* by Elmer Cranton, MD. A new technique of chelating therapy that works. Especially directed toward those with heart and circulatory disease.

7. *Quantum Healing* by Deepak Chopra, MD. This man has contributed his life to helping reverse the illness of many. He has several books in print on mind and body connection, and all are worthy of your time. He is one of my wife's favorite authors for restoring health. What's good for her is good for me.

8. *Miracle Cures, Stop Aging Now!* and *Food: Your Miracle Medicine* by Jean Carper. She presents scientific evidence of the effectiveness of natural remedies and relates them to many self-cures. Making notes in your books as you read helps when needed. Another real gem of a site is 1cure4cancer.com.

9. *Fit for Life* by Harvey and Marilyn Diamond. Contains general information on eating and should be a must on your list.

10. I saved the best book for last. *The Cure for All Advanced Cancers* by Hulda Clark, PhD, ND. This book is not about remission; it is about eliminating the disease. Her success rate is 95 percent. The establishment would like to close her down, but the proof is evident and documented. She obtained her doctorate degree at the University of Minnesota then performed government-sponsored research for ten years at Indiana University.

Later she earned a naturopathy degree in 1979. This woman deserves the Nobel Prize for love and compassion for mankind, not persecution by the establishment. Her Zapper is one of the finest and a monument to her dedication to stamping out disease. She is a brilliant scientist (microbiologist) and servant of mankind. If you don't buy any of the above books, buy this one while it is still available in print. Hopefully, you won't need it; but it is good information to have, and you may be able to help others who do need it.

Now for the Web sites that give information and updates as to what is going on in the world of health. Most sites have something to sell, but many just want to reveal the injustice and travesty against the human race. In all new information, you have to be aware of the intention and motivation behind the profound claims. Please do not believe anything you read without documenting it for yourself as words are cheap and easy to come by. Without substance and meaning, words are platitudes to be thrown to the wind. Ask God for discernment.

Tools for Healing

1. **Drhuldaclark.org** – You will find her Web page under her name and a list of her books as mentioned before. She also lists suggested herbs that have been tested for purity. You may get on her mailing list as I am. She needs our support because she is on a crusade to save the world from ignorance when it comes to health. She is a strong-willed and brilliant woman who loves her work and is dedicated to bringing healing to a world of ignorance.

2. **Drkelley.com** – You will find his whole book on the Net, and you can download it for nothing. What a great story of his self-recovery from pancreatic cancer and how this man went on to help hundreds in his inconspicuous small office in Texas near Dallas. He was a dentist who converted his life to exposing the truth about cancer

treatment. He is now seventy-five, and his family continues his work with him.

3. **Gatewaytohealth.com "All diseases are curable, but not all people"** – In this site you will find a wonderful and inspiring group exchanging ideas and experiences online. You can get sincere help from concerned people who enjoy exchanging their personal experiences with others in need of help. Lots of good, reliable testimonies.

4. **Sotainstruments.com** – This is the place to purchase the Zapper by Bob Beck. They have all the information that you need if you decide to order a Zapper. It is my lifeline to good health and an inexpensive investment. Type in the word *Zapper* on the Internet, and you will find many different kinds at various prices.

5. **Don Croft's "The Terminator"** – This is a must for your health (zapper16@earthlink.net). He has had real success with it in Africa against AIDS. Read deeply into this technology as it could be your salvation against the possibility of unknown terrorist biological warfare.

6. **h2o2-4u.com** – They have documented the great medicinal uses of this natural product for our health. Look it up for yourself as there is a bundle of information on the Net. I rinse my mouth out every morning with HP to keep infections at bay.

7. **Colloidalsilver.com** – Colloidal silver is a must to research on the "beast." Don't buy it when you can make it so cheap. Buying a machine is reasonable and a sound investment for maintenance of good health. This is the media's best-kept secret for all-around health support except on the Internet. I use this every day of my life as an immune system booster. Also, look it up on "The Gateway to Health."

8. Black walnut-wormwood-cloves combination is a must in my medicine cabinet for me and my dog. This is a proven method that has had tremendous success in killing parasites in our bodies.

After coming back from Central America, my wife and I both were infested, and they played havoc with our immune systems. We experienced all kinds of symptoms such as bloating, indigestion, mucous buildup, respiratory ailments . . . and the list goes on. So it didn't take a rocket scientist to let us know that our immune systems were working double time. By reading and applying the process of controlling these invaders in our bodies, we were able to overcome all symptoms in a short period of time. Look to curezone. org and certainly drhuldaclark.org for maintaining control over the documented 550-plus species of parasites that inhabit our bodies as their home. It is an ongoing battle as we keep re-infesting our bodies. I purchase most of my support minerals and vitamins from Dr. Clark's Web site as they check the product for purity and make sure the potency of ingredients are as stated on the labels. Unfortunately, many health food supplements are not up to standard and, in fact, fall short of purity and contain a lot of superfluous additives. I also check with my local health food store and ask for the better brands that maintain top standards.

Doctors of the future will give no medicine but will interest his patients in the care of the human frame, in diet, and in the cause and prevention of disease.

– Thomas Edison

Summary

D O NOT GIVE up on this earthly journey as so many of us seniors are willing to do. Because we harbor a wonderful, secure belief in God, we are the only light bearers left in this world of madness. Our generation still projects *love and hope* into the insanity and despair that is being propagated in this so-called modern civilization. Survive, my dear readers, as a living testimony to that love of freedom and peace that our nation once projected throughout the world. *Live the rest our your life with that divine purpose.*

If I got a little carried away with the importance of this information and the politics related to it, blame my desire to stand up and be accounted for (and ADHD). I publish this book with a prayer that the information it offers might reach receptive souls and make a real and lasting difference in their lives. I also offer that you share this information with others that may be receptive to its message. My main interest, as I'm sure you're aware of by now, is to combat and destroy the media mind-set that opposes commonsense healing. What will make my day is if this little book can, in some small way, help humans discard old and ineffective ideas of seeking quick cures from the establishment when real and perpetual healing is within us.

I have offered some of the major Web sites and books that I have found to be reliable and applicable to sustaining my own optimum health. What you do with this information is within your own discernment to determine the credibility and practicality of its message and how it can be applied to your life. May God grant you wisdom to make the life-sustaining decisions that will have a permanent impact on you during this great and wonderful journey through life. God bless you all, and seek peace and comfort in his love.

The most gratifying moment in any person's life must be when
he has given life-preserving assistance to a receptive soul that was
on the verge of desperation and destruction.

– Ty Hardin

A letter to the readers who has suffered through this feeble attempt to express very important and vital information.

This is an invitation for all souls to get involved in helping me get the best healing programs out to those concerned readers. I welcome any and all additions and other information that will enhance and improve the quality and reliability of this information. The little book is on my computer and can be altered with every new printing. With your help and my wife's, who supports me with love and spelling, we can continue to keep this open book up-to-date and inspire others to meet the challenges that are before us. We can meet the reality of the end of our free society.

His chosen are being prepared for these end-times and the return of our Lord. My firm conviction is we are going to see much devastation and disasters before that promised return of our Lord comes to place. A great cleansing of our land is in the process as we have neglected our first love and followed after the beast. Get prepared for his return and prepare your lives to meet whatever disaster the Lord has in store for you. Continue searching the "beast" while we keep upgrading the text offered in our little e-book along with adding new vital information as it's revealed and documented to me. This is a work in progress until I'm called home. I will encourage you to send all your personal testimonies, order books and pictures, and comments to my e-mail address (ty.bronco@gmail.com); and I will address your offerings with respect and prayer. Thank you again and keep the faith as our Lord's hidden army will prevail in these trying times as people are waking up all over America as to their government's priorities. As far as I am concerned, it couldn't happen at a better time as it will help us get it right the next time.

As I go to press, Russia is fighting to keep its allies protected from our war machine that's placing missile bases all over Europe, intimidating their sovereignty. We are jeopardizing the world peace with our threat of an atomic holocaust. The world is tired of our war machine intimidating and intruding on their freedoms. They have a God-given right to live without the fear of being bombed into oblivion. When are we going to be content with living on our own soil, taking care of our citizens, and seeking a peaceful existence with all mankind?

A TRIBUTE TO MY FELLOW THESPIANS

The following photo gallery is dedicated to the actors ,actresses, stuntmen and crew with whom I was privileged to work, many of whom are now deceased. Without their contribution, my career would have been short-lived.

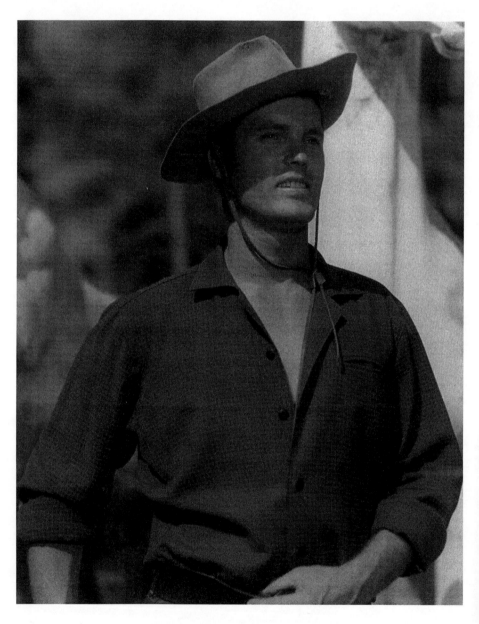

Ty, as Bronco, in production shot

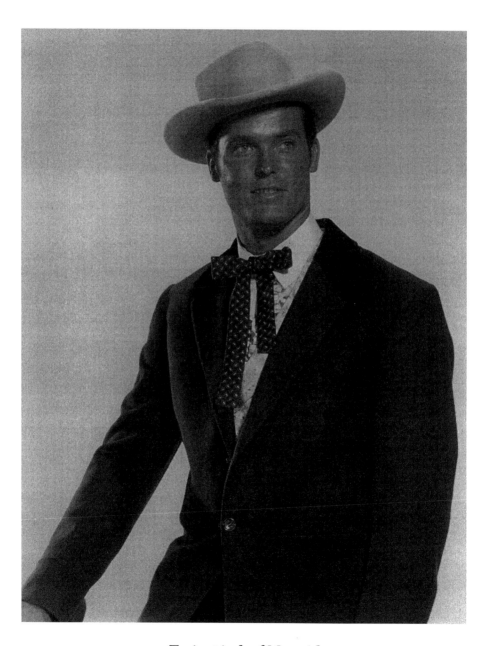

Ty, in episode of Maverick

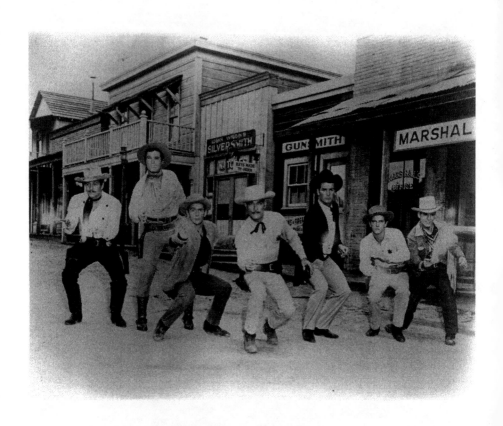

Warner Brothers Television Cowboys
L to R: Wade Preston, Colt 45
Ty Hardin, Bronco Layne
Jack Kelly, Maverick
John Russell, Lawman
James Garner, Maverick
Peter Brown, Lawman
Will Hutchins, Sugarfoot

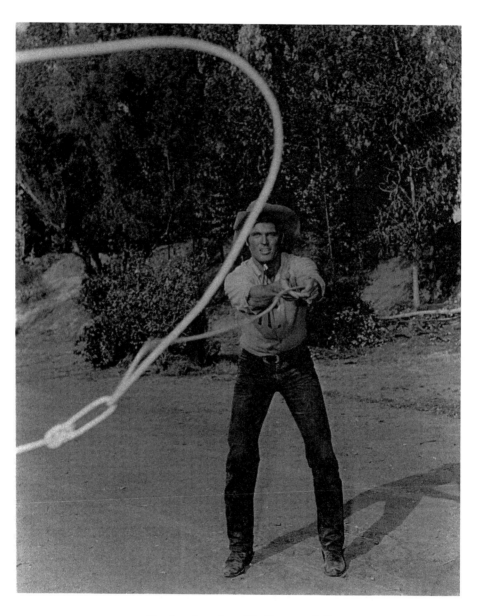

Production shot, Ty "just ropin"

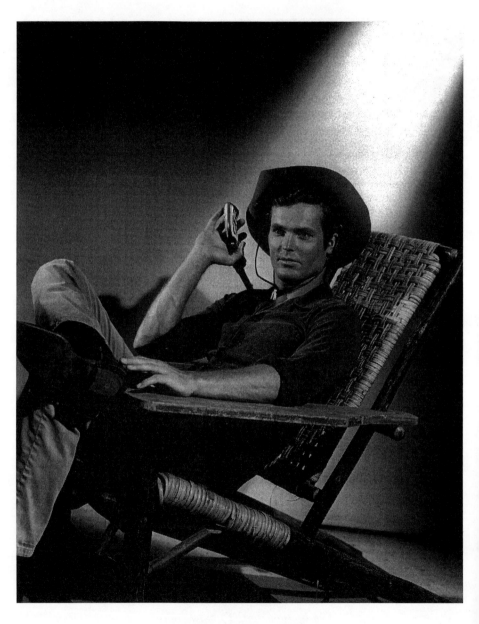

Ty, "a quiet moment"

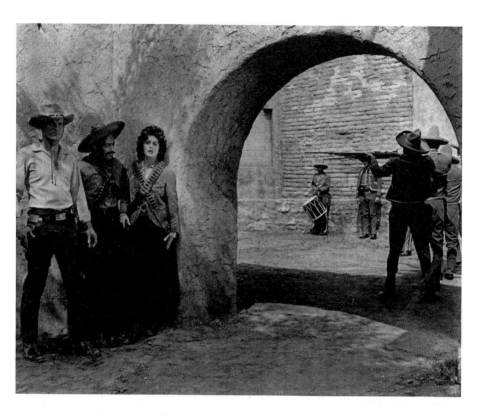

Bronco with Faith Domerque and Carlos Romero
in "La Rubia"

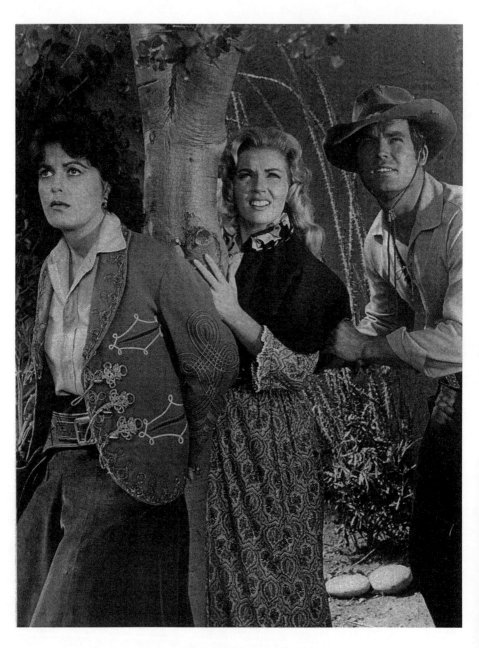

Bronco episode with Faith Domergue and Joan O'Brien
in "La Rubia"

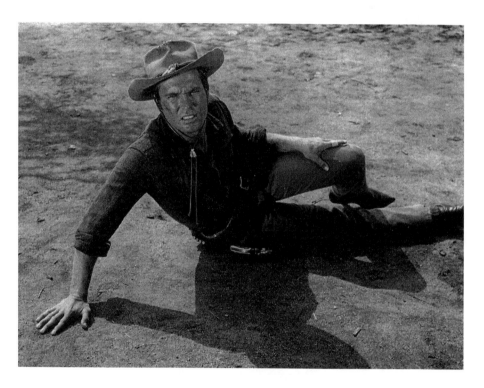

Bronco "bucked off"

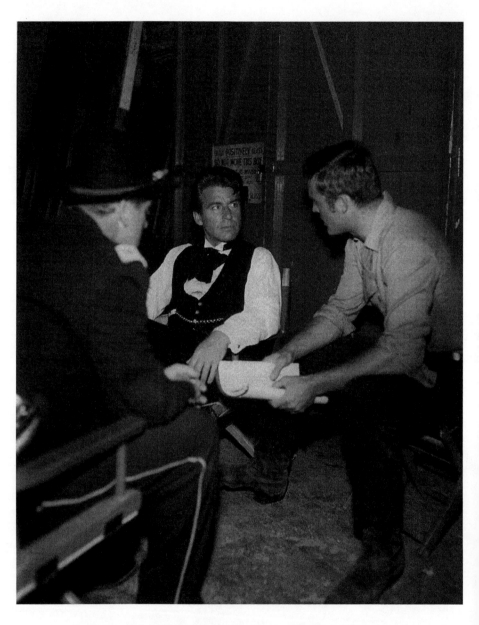

Bronco with Efrem Zimbalist, Jr. in "Prince of Darkness"

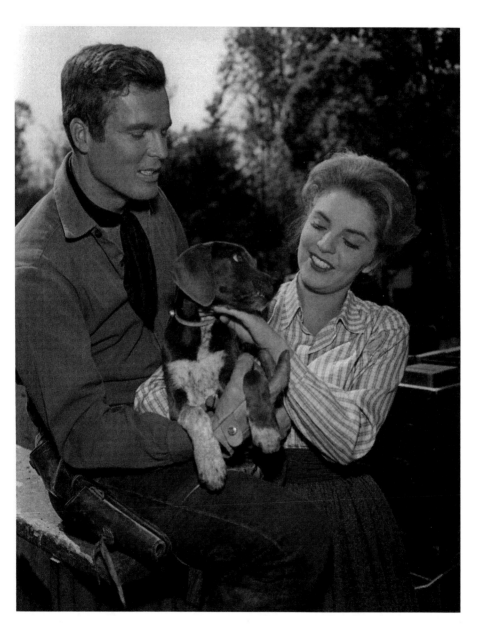

Bronco & Susan Seaforth in "Then the Mountain"

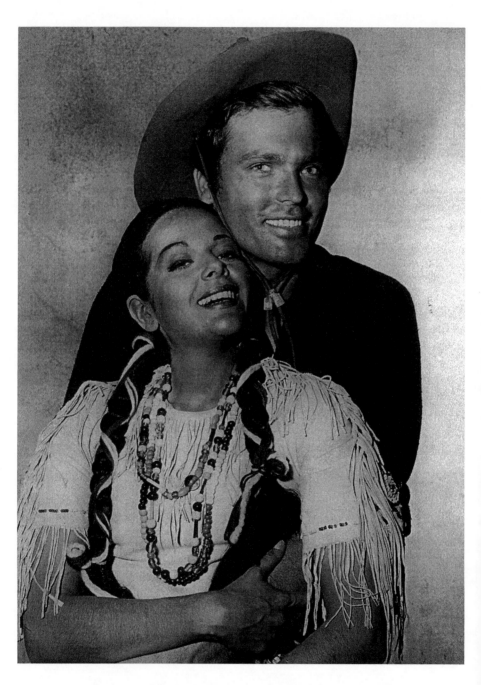

Bronco with Yvette Dugay in "School for Cowards"

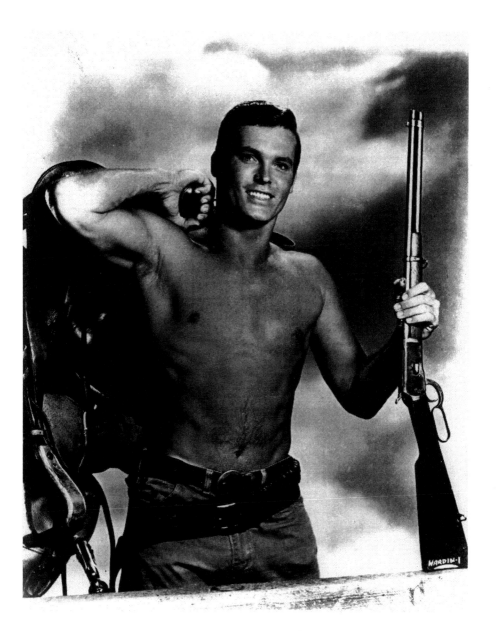

"Beefcake shot" for Jack Warner

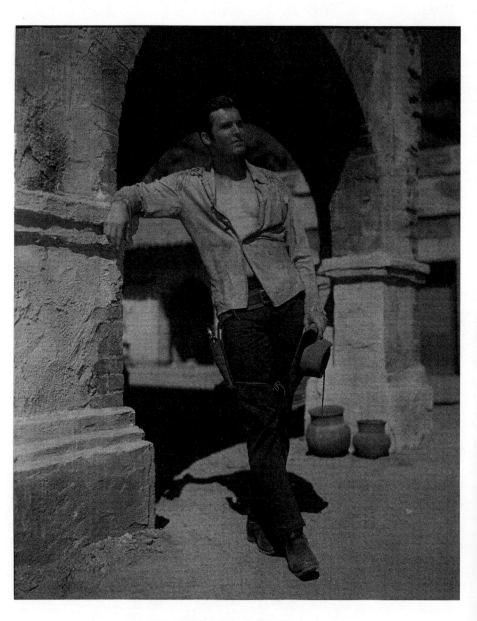

Ty, production shot at mission for "La Rubia"

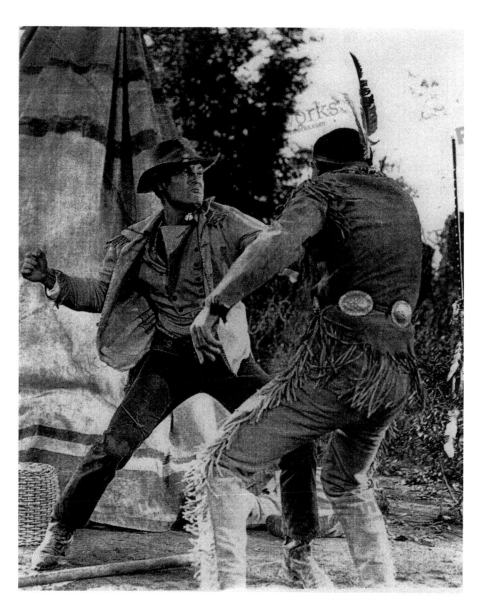

Bronco fighting with Yakima

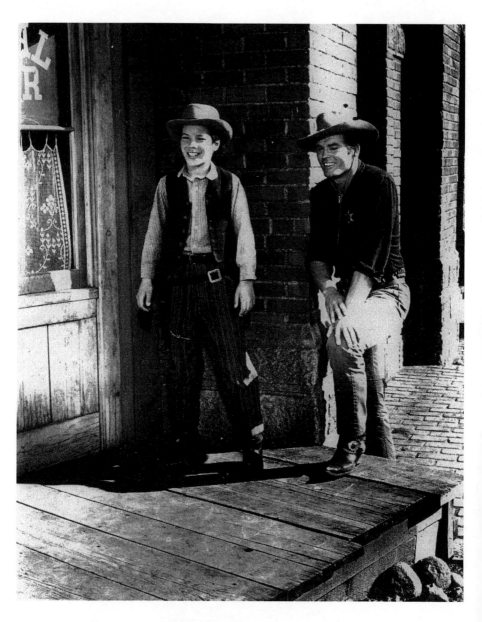

Bronco with young costar

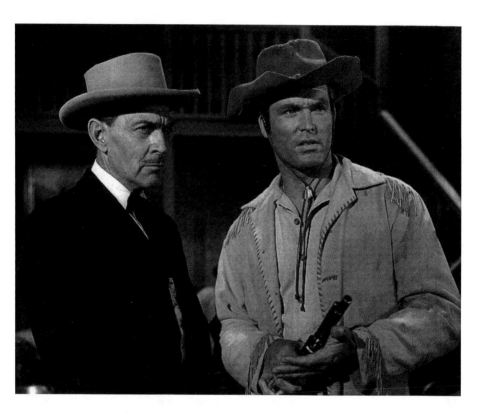

Bronco with Kent Taylor

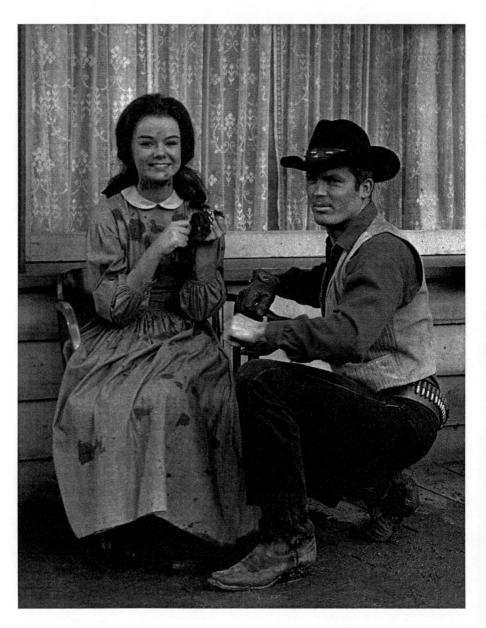

Bronco and Anna Capri in "The Town That Lived & Died"

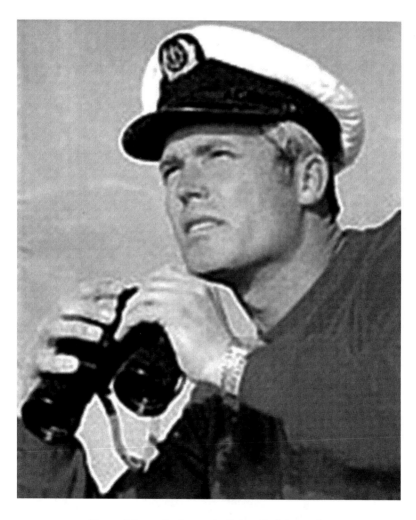

Ty as Moss Andrews in Riptide/Australia

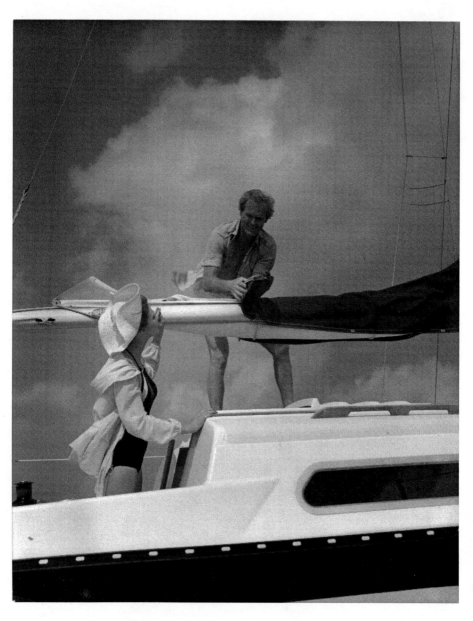

Sailing in Riptide with Aussie Beauty

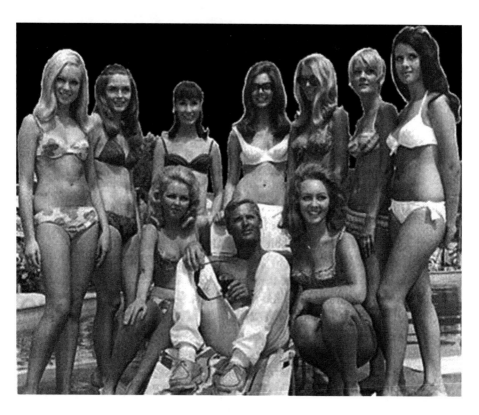

The Beauties from Riptide Series

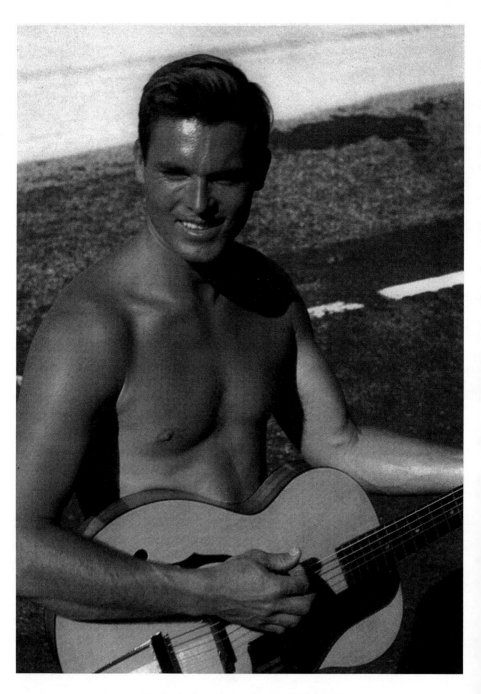

Ty "strumming on Sorrento Beach"

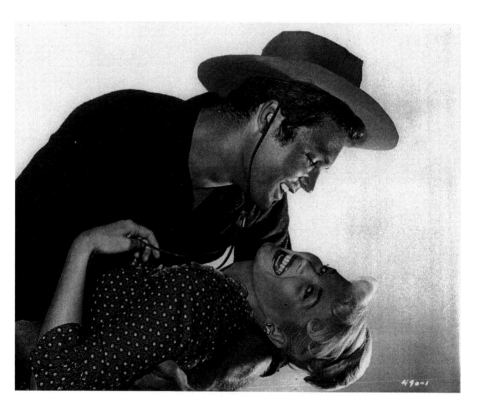

Production shot of Ty and Dorothy Provine

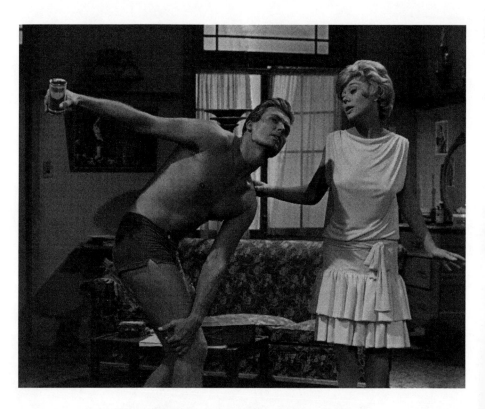

Ty and Glynis John in the Chapman Report

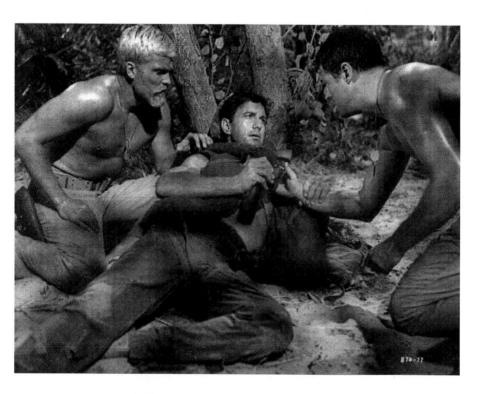

Ty, Cliff Robertson and Robert Culp in PT109

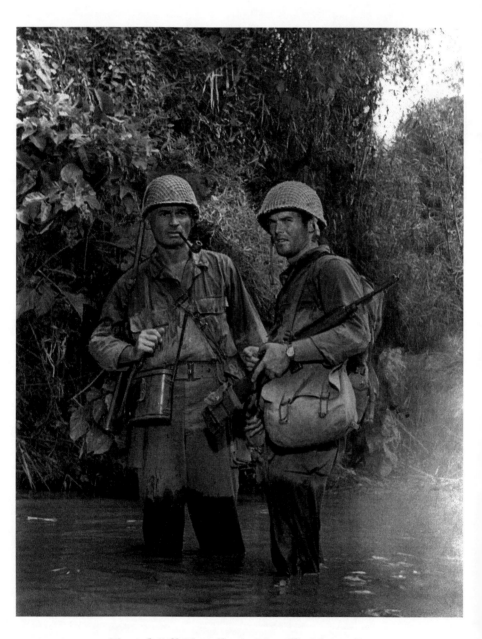

Ty and Jeff Chandler in Merrill's Marauders

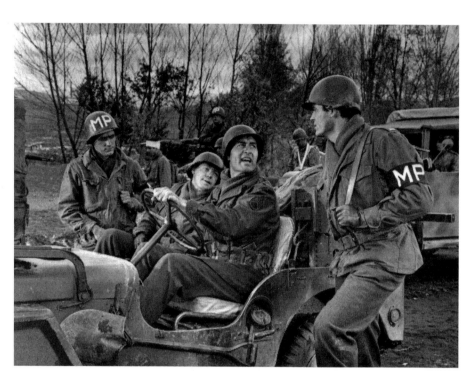

*Ty Hardin as the German Spy posing as an American
in Battle of the Bulge, pictured here with
George Montgomery and James McArthur*

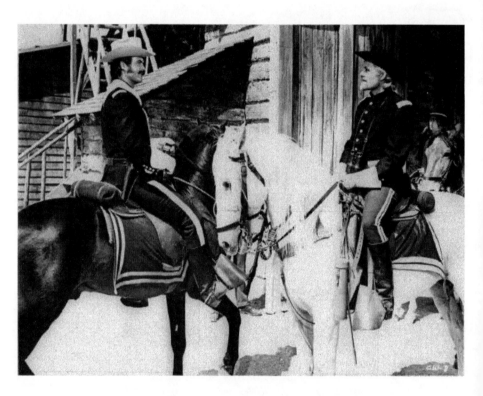

Ty and Robert Shaw in Custer of the West

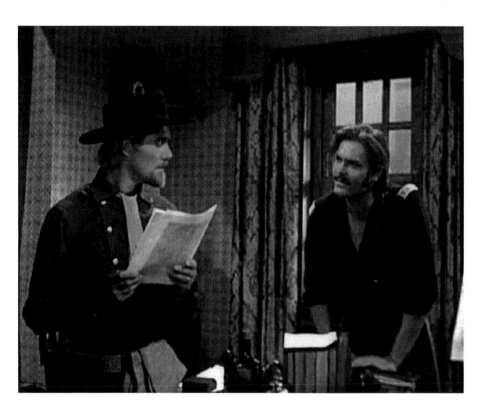

Ty and Robert Shaw in Custer of the West

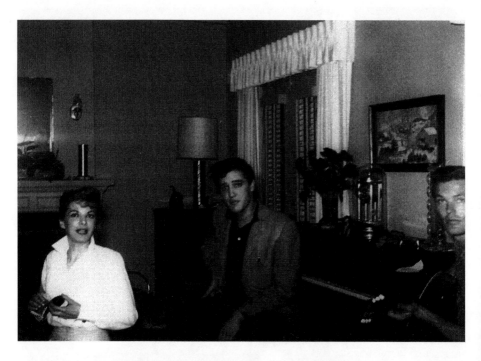

Actress, Jan Shepard (notably of "Paradise, Hawaiian Style with the "King", at her birthday party, pictured with Elvis and me on the right

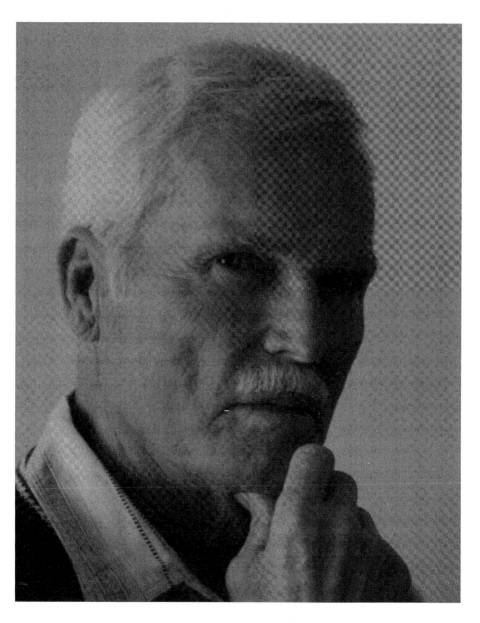

Recent photo of Ty

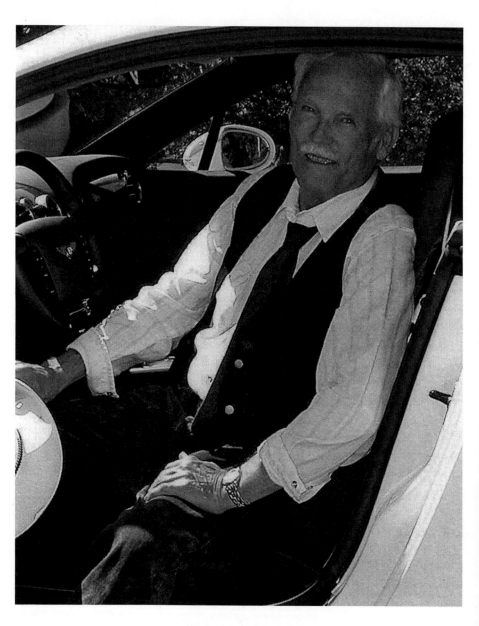

Ty on his way to work

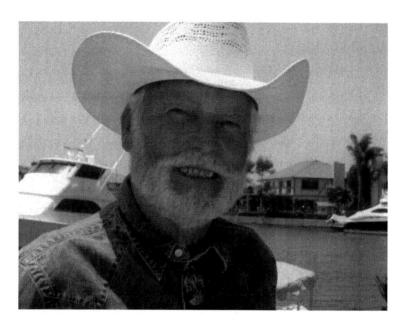

Ty on the waterfront

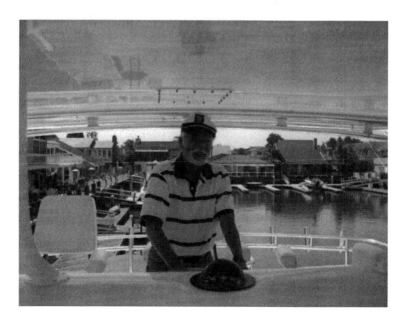

Captain Ty coming into the dock

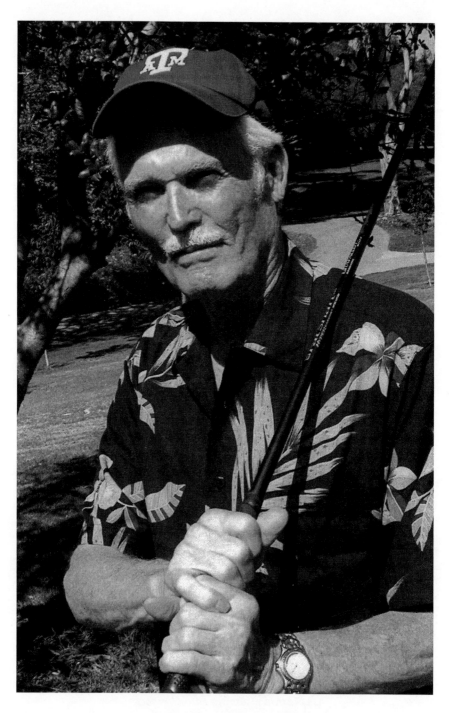

Ty, just putting around

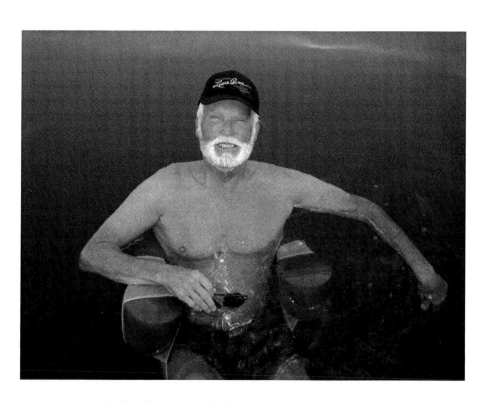

Hydrotherapy at Shadow Lake, Indio, California

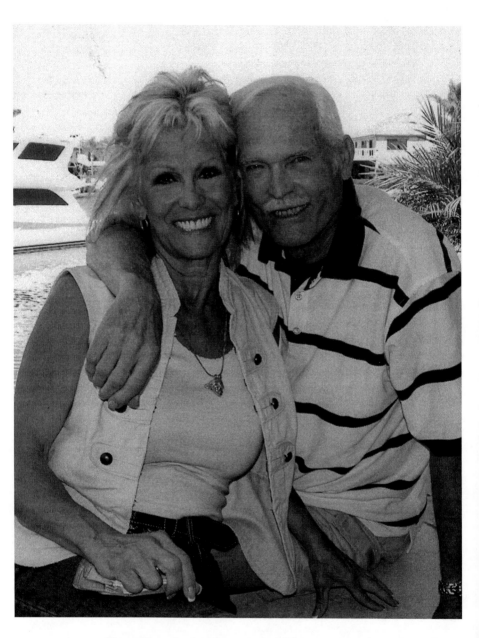

Ty with wife, Caroline, in Huntington Harbor